Addictions can be cured

The
Treatment
of Drug Addiction
by Neuro-Electric
Stimulation

An interim report
by
Margaret A Patterson
MBE, MBChB, FRCSE

Lion Publishing

LION PUBLISHING
121 *High St, Berkhamsted, Herts*

First edition 1975

International Standard Book Number 0 85648 041 x

Printed in Great Britain
by Hazell Watson and Viney, Ltd., Aylesbury, Bucks

Contents

	Preface	7
1	**Discovery of Treatment** *Initial encounters with acupuncture • Acupuncture anaesthesia in Hong Kong.*	9
2	**Background to Treatment** *Chinese medical tradition • Acupuncture theory • Acupuncture anaesthesia theory • Electro-analgesia in the West • Neural effects and chemical changes • Electro-anaesthesia • Electro-sleep.*	15
3	**Development of Treatment** *Experimentation in Hong Kong • Official discouragement in Hong Kong • Successful treatment of status asthmaticus • Importance of the electrical factor in stimulation.*	30
4	**Associated Medical/Electronic Treatments** *Addiction and electrical stimulation • Epilepsy and stimulation • The cerebellum and stimulation • Pain and stimulation • Bio feedback and brain rhythms • Post-operative stimulation • The 'Great Bordeaux Magnetic Machine' • Cerebral palsy, spasticity and stimulation • The 'Cooper Brain Pacemaker' • Possible structural change after stimulation • Tissue regeneration and stimulation.*	38
5	**Present State of Treatment** *Electrical significance of acupuncture points • Stimulation of animals • Importance of form of electrical current • Possible enduring neuro-chemical changes • Electrical activity in damaged nerves • Different reactions in electrical stimulation with different drugs • Pocket-size stimulator for home use • Frequency range in various conditions • Intensity of treatment • Duration of treatment • Treatment of pain • Summary of investigations • Side effects.*	53
6	**Rehabilitation Treatments: Some Spiritual Aspects** *Relationship between drugs and the occult • Doctors and the middle-aged to blame • Drug dependence and drug addiction • Drugs and their mystical effects • Some significant treatments of addiction • The necessity for spiritual values.*	70
7	**Appendices** 1. *Multi-purpose electro-therapeutic apparatus for Chinese acupuncture points* • 2. *Opium and heroin addiction: material and result* • 3. *Acupuncture and electro-stimulation for asthmatic attacks* • 4. *The Shackman-Patterson electrical stimulator.*	87

'Incredible phenomena are attached to the cure; medicine is powerless against them, beyond making the padded cell look like a hotel-room and demanding of the doctor or nurse patience, attendance and sensitivity . . .

'I therefore became an opium addict again because the doctors who cure—one should really say, quite simply, who purge—do not seek to cure the troubles which first cause the addiction . . .'

'After the cure. The worst moment, the worst danger. Health with this void and an immense sadness. The doctors honestly hand you over to suicide.'

'Now that I am cured, I feel empty, poor, heart-broken and ill.'

Jean Cocteau

Preface

This book is compiled from the substance of several talks and articles, and is only intended as an interim report describing my investigations for the informed layman, or as a guideline for professional colleagues who are interested in developments in this new field.

It is not my intention to publish anything professionally definitive until I have completed the present stage of my two-year period of research.

However, I hope this gives sufficient indication of the possibilities to encourage others to pursue or expand their own investigations, and to make a contribution to the growing amount of significant material in the field of neuro-electric stimulation.

The list of books and articles, from both Chinese and Western sources, which formed the background reading for the following outline is too voluminous to list in a popular book of this kind, but I wish to record my particular appreciation to Dr H. L. Wen, Dr Felix Mann, Professor Patrick D. Wall, Dr Robert D. Becker, the Editor of the Asian Journal of Modern Medicine for permission to reproduce material from Volume 9, April and June 1973, and most of all to Dr Irving S. Cooper for his unfailing encouragement and advice. Finally, I owe a special debt of gratitude to Robert Stigwood whose personal interest and research grant made this work possible.

Words are inadequate to express what I owe to my husband's inspiration and practical help.

M. A. Patterson, MBE, MBChB, FRCSE

Chapter One
Discovery of Treatment

If there is a single figure most responsible for the recent upsurge of interest in acupuncture in the West it is the *New York Times*' columnist and Vice-President, James Reston. Shortly after his arrival in Peking with President Nixon in 1972, Reston developed appendicitis. His appendix was removed by surgeons at the Anti-Imperial Hospital under conventional anaesthesia but afterwards he permitted an acupuncturist to apply needles to his elbow and legs to relieve post-surgical pain. He wrote:

'There was a noticeable relaxation of pressure and distension within an hour, and no recurrence of the problem thereafter . . .'

US physicians began taking acupuncture seriously shortly afterwards, when a group of their most eminent colleagues, including Boston heart specialist Dr Paul Dudley White and New York ear surgeon Dr Samuel Rosen, toured Chinese hospitals and watched fully conscious patients undergo major surgery with nothing more than acupuncture to anaesthetise them.

The operations observed by the astonished doctors included partial removal of the stomach, excision of a brain tumour and the removal of an ovarian cyst. Dr Rosen reported on his return to the US:

'My colleagues and I have seen the past, and it works.'

Initial encounters with acupuncture

I first became interested in acupuncture in 1963 when my husband was assisting a journalist colleague, Guy Wint, to edit the *Asia Handbook*.[1] Guy Wint at that time had suffered a severe stroke

1 Published by Blond and Briggs, 1965 and Penguin Books, 1969.

which left him partially paralysed in body and disordered in speech. He was reduced to frustrating inactivity and continuous pain requiring heavy sedation. He heard of Dr Felix Mann, a Consultant in my old hospital, St James's, Balham, who practised acupuncture, and asked if I would discuss the treatment with him.

A few years later, in his book, *The Third Killer*,[2] Guy Wint described his experience of a variety of treatments in different parts of the world, and declared:

'By far the most rewarding of these experiments was with Chinese acupuncture. It was surprising that this was so because at first the doctor who practised it—Dr Felix Mann, from Cambridge, trained in Western medicine—asserted that it would do little for strokes, and tried to dissuade me from having this administration. Later I discovered in a Chinese handbook that the Chinese themselves use it in such cases, but they recognize that a stroke is altogether a very serious matter, and a cure is not very likely . . .'

I was so impressed by Guy Wint's improvement, and by that of several others whom I sent to Dr Mann for treatment, that when I arrived in Hong Kong in 1964 to take up an appointment as Head of Surgery with the Tung Wah Group of Hospitals, I decided to have the acupuncture treatment for my own migraine. I had been a sufferer from migraine for thirty years, with three three-day attacks almost every two weeks, only made tolerable by large doses of drugs.

I was introduced by a mutual friend to a Chinese acupuncturist. He was a film distributor, not a doctor, but he had studied and practised acupuncture all his life, first in China and later in France, and was well-informed on the subject of anatomy. He told me that I would have to have three courses of treatment over a period of three months.

The first month's treatments were quite dramatically successful. Both the frequency and the intensity of the attacks was reduced by 95 per cent. In the second month, with the needles placed in

2 Published by Chatto and Windus, 1965.

the corner of the eye in addition to other sites, improvement was only 50 per cent. In the third month, attacks were as severe as ever and the needling, which was at first painless, had become very painful.

However, the same acupuncturist later treated my husband very successfully for an arthritic knee caused by a damaged cartilage. The cartilage trouble was the legacy of an old football injury which began to be very painful and caused him sleepless nights. I arranged an appointment with an orthopaedic surgeon colleague who established by X-ray that there were osteoarthritic changes in the knee. He gave my husband cortisone injections. Six weeks later the pain was back, as bad—and unbearable—as ever. Yet after two half-hour treatments with needles and electrical stimulation by the acupuncturist, the pain disappeared. Almost three years have passed since then and it has not returned.

Striking as these and other personal observations were, they were really only conversation pieces, items of bizarre oriental exotica, compared to the phenomena that confronted me at the end of 1972. It was the implication and potential of these phenomena which took me out of the surgery I had loved and practised for 25 years. It started, strangely enough, on my birthday, 9 November 1972.

Following Samuel Rosen and Paul Dudley White, other doctors visited China and were equally impressed by developments in Chinese medicine. Dr E. Grey Dimond, provost of the University of Missouri Medical School in Kansas City, was one. In the *Journal of the American Medical Association* he listed the advantages the Chinese had found in acupuncture anaesthesia:

'It is absolutely safe; there is no interruption of the patient's hydration. The patient can still receive fluid and foods. There is no post-operative nausea and vomiting. The method is convenient and readily available.'

But the Chinese doctors told their Western colleagues that despite trying acupuncture anaesthesia on over 500,000 patients, with a 90 per cent success rate,[3] they could still offer no adequate

3 *Acupuncture Anaesthesia*, Foreign Languages Press, Peking.

explanation. They used acupuncture because it worked. The leading theory inside China was that acupuncture as an anaesthetic involved 'neuro-physiological phenomena, and that basically the twirling needles were thought to send an impulse to the brain that reduced the electrical activity there which would otherwise register pain'.

Acupuncture anaesthesia in Hong Kong

One of my Chinese colleagues in the Tung Wah Group of Hospitals was Dr H. L. Wen, a well-known Hong Kong neurosurgeon who was Consultant to the Neuro-Surgical Unit. He was extremely interested in the possibilities of using acupuncture anaesthesia in some of his brain operations. On his return to Hong Kong, after a month's visit to China to study the techniques, he asked me as Head of Surgery to select some patients willing to have acupuncture anaesthesia for their operations instead of the orthodox nitrous oxide. Dr Wen's senior assistant, Dr Stanley Y. C. Cheung, was one of my own trainee surgeons who had assisted me before sitting for his Edinburgh Fellowship and doing advanced training at the Edinburgh Neuro-Surgical Unit.

It was while we were experimenting with the acupuncture anaesthesia that we discovered we were curing drug addicts serendipitously. Unknown to us, some of the patients had been on drugs—opium, heroin, morphine, nicotine and alcohol—for a number of years. Some had been heavily addicted for many years to doses far in excess of anything tolerated in the West. And they spontaneously volunteered the information that in the few weeks since we had started needling them they had lost their desire for their drugs, cigarettes or alcohol.

It was Dr Wen who first suggested a possible connection between acupunctural stimulation operating on the autonomic nervous system and the withdrawal symptoms of drug addiction. He then asked me to look out specially for drug addicts among the patients, and we began to keep detailed notes of their responses, with increasing interest.

In February 1973, a well-known US neuro-physiologist and neuro-surgeon, Dr Irving Cooper, visited Hong Kong and gave a lecture to the Tung Wah Group of Hospitals. Dr Cooper, from St Barnabas Hospital for Chronic Diseases in New York, became internationally known as a pioneer of several new brain operations for involuntary movement disorders (including Parkinson's disease) and techniques in cryogenic surgery. At his lecture Dr Cooper revealed that he might have discovered yet another medical advance—a possible means of curing epileptics and spastics by implanting electrodes in the brain by surgery and then stimulating them by means of a receiver implanted in the chest, and a pocket transmitter. His theory was that prosthetic stimulation of the cerebellum may gradually recondition reflex functioning of some brain circuits or lead to enduring neuro-chemical changes.

This was deeply challenging to me. If it could be established that there was some connection between what Dr Cooper was investigating and our own discovery of the effects of electro-acupuncture it opened up some tremendous possibilities. Dr Cooper himself was interested. He affirmed that some present theories about the physiology of the brain might have to be reconsidered in the light of this. And he added that most recent researches by neuro-surgeons suggested that evidence was emerging that electrical stimulation reconditioned circuits such as the reticular formation so that, in conditions formerly believed incurable, there was progressive improvement the longer the treatment was carried on.

Later, on reflection, an idea suddenly struck me. What if the Chinese, without knowing about electricity, had yet stumbled on another profound discovery several thousand years before? Acupuncture might well be a form of electrical stimulation to correct a metabolic imbalance, and the very recent electro-acupunctural stimulation simply a more intense form of the original 'twirling' practice. In that case the acupuncture points would be less important in the drug addiction cures than the electric stimulation of the nerve pathways to the brain—occurring in some way yet to be discovered.

Chapter Two

Background to Treatment

Chinese herbal medicine is over four thousand years old, the first pharmacy book, the *P'en T'sao*, being published by the Emperor Shen Nung in 2737 BC. This book listed 365 herbs as 'superior, mediocre or inferior'. The now famous *Ephedrine*, brought to the notice of the West by a Dr K. K. Chen in 1926, was listed in the *P'en T'sao* as 'ma huang' and has been used by Chinese doctors to treat asthma for four thousand years.

Chinese medical tradition

The *Huang Ti Nei Ching Su Wen*, or *The Yellow Emperor's Classic of Internal Medicine*, is the earliest extant medical classic of China, written between the 8th and 5th centuries BC. It consists of 18 volumes covering a great variety of subjects, including the theory of diseases and their etiology, diagnosis and treatment.

In the book, man is seen as a microcosm of the universe and subject to the same tensions as nature itself. The immutable course of nature, the Tao, was believed to act through two opposing and unifying forces, the Yin—negative, passive and femine—and the Yang—positive, active and masculine. In a normal person the two forces are in balance and assist the vital energy—called *chi*—to circulate to all parts of the body via a network of 14 channels or 'meridians', each connected to an important internal organ or junction to which it branches. Obstruction (deficiency) and outpouring (excess) in the circulation of the *chi* causes an imbalance of the two forces and thus results in disease.

Chinese traditional medicine and philosophy is based on the interpretation and conception of *chi*. It was believed that all things, animate or inanimate, possess an inherent factor of energy;

this stabilizes the chemical composition of matter, and when this matter is broken down—as in nuclear fission, for example—energy is released. Water and ice have the same chemical formula, yet when one changes into the other, energy, in some form or other, is liberated. Man is made of matter but he has life also. Thus he has two sources of energy: the electrical energy which is generated as a result of the biochemical and biophysical changes in his cells; and the living energy he has inherited by his birth.[1]

The Chinese phrase for medicine consists of four radicals, or symbols, in two characters: one meaning a cavity with an arrow inside it; and the other meaning a knife or instrument, and alcohol. Chinese scholars interpret the phrase to mean that an arrow has created a wound and that a knife or some instrument is needed to extract it, with alcohol applied to treat it. So, in spite of later speculations and often absurd theories as to the causation and cure of diseases there was always a rational, semi-scientific and dignified practice of empirical treatment based on the accumulated knowledge of centuries and derived from acute observation by intelligent men of integrity.

Acupuncture (from the Latin *acus*, 'needle', and *pungere*, 'to sting') has been used in China in one form or another for some five thousand years. Legend has it that the practice evolved after a soldier, struck by an arrow in battle, noticed a sensation of numbness distant from the wound.

But the practice of acupuncture developed in conjunction with moxibustion, or the burning of the herb mogwart at or near the appropriate sites of the body. So as the Chinese name for acupuncture, *chen-chiu* ('needle and heat') implies, it usually incorporated both practices. Acupuncture and moxibustion, combined with the use of herbs, breathing and therapeutic massage, still constitute the core of traditional Chinese medicine.

In *The Yellow Emperor's Classic of Internal Medicine* there were detailed descriptions of the various needles used in acu-

1 Dr Louis Moss, a Western expert on acupuncture, has stated (*Acupuncture and You*, Dell Publishing Co., 1972): 'It may well be that this force (*chi*) is an electrical potential emanating from the minutest cells in the body by their biochemical and biophysical exchanges.'

puncture and the various parts of the body where they could be used most effectively. During the following two and a half millennia many hundreds of acupuncture points were recorded, each one named after its discoverer, and many theories were advanced to explain how and why it worked as it did.

Acupuncture theory

The most widely accepted modern theory, as we have already mentioned, is that the prick of the needle at certain precisely defined points on the skin stimulates specific nerves which transmit electrical impulses to the spinal cord and lower centres of the brain and thence to the diseased area. Nerves are supplied to every part of the body, no matter how small, and every millimetre of it is under the direct control of one nerve or a group of nerves. They control nearly all processes going on in the body. When stimulated, some nerves will increase the movement of the intestines, others retard it. Some will increase, others retard, the flow of the digestive juices. Similarly, certain nerves can increase or decrease the rate of the heart, determine the expansion or contraction of blood vessels, and so on.

Dr Felix Mann, the leading Western authority on acupuncture, has written:

'The nervous system can be compared to the electronic control apparatus of some complex machine, like a telephone exchange or an automatic pilot. The art of acupuncture depends on knowing precisely which nerve to stimulate in a given disease. It sounds as simple as knowing which keys to press on a typewriter in order to spell your own name. In fact, however, a considerable amount of knowledge is needed before acupuncture can be practised satisfactorily . . .'[2]

Before the West, with its recently developed system of scientific medicine, made an impact on China, the health of the nation depended on the practitioners of this traditional Chinese medicine. The Chinese doctor rarely practised surgery, and, under the Manchu dynasty, he was not allowed to do so.

2 *Acupuncture: Cure of Many Diseases*, William Heinemann Medical Books, 1972.

With the introduction of Western medicine in China, traditional medicine in general and acupuncture in particular began to fall into disrepute as being non-scientific. In 1822 the Great Imperial Board ordered the virtual abandonment of acupuncture on ethical grounds. Chinese intellectuals educated in Western missionary schools came to regard Chinese medicine as old-fashioned and a hindrance to the modernization and development of their country. In 1929 the Kuomintang Government banned the practice of traditional Chinese medicine, including acupuncture.

But despite this, the ordinary Chinese citizen continued to believe in and use acupuncture and traditional medicine. Accurate statistics on the number of physicians practising in China in 1950 when the Communist Government took over control are not available, but estimates vary from 10,000 to 40,000 to care for 550 million people. That may sound like one doctor to 15,000 people but in fact the doctors mostly practised in urban areas. Eighty per cent of the population, living in rural areas, had virtually no benefit from the Western-trained doctors. They relied on an estimated 400,000 traditional doctors, using treatment by herbal medicines and acupuncture for the relief of pain.

The present Chinese Communist Government, after taking office in 1949, rectified this situation by introducing the Maoist policy of 'walking on both feet'. Mao Tse-Tung set out four concepts of health care:

1. to serve the workers and peasants and soldiers;
2. to put prevention first;
3. to unite Western and traditional Chinese medicine; and
4. to co-ordinate medical campaigns with mass movements.

They built new hospitals, rehabilitated old ones and greatly multiplied medical school enrolment. At the same time they increased the number of nurses, midwives and assistant doctors, and developed a new type of para-medical called 'the barefoot doctor', 'worker doctor' and 'Red Guard doctor'. These were peasants, factory-workers or soldiers, given approximately three months training and subsequent on-the-job training in the provision of basic health care. The integration of traditional and Western medicine was repeatedly stressed by Chairman Mao who stated:

'Chinese medicine and pharmacology are a great treasure house; efforts should be made to explore them and raise them to higher levels.'

Reactionary doctors were urged to abandon conservative prejudices, to accept new knowledge, study science and co-operate with their Western-type counterparts.

Acupuncture anaesthesia theory

Acupuncture was first used for surgical anaesthesia in China in 1958. The first successful acupuncture anaesthesia was for tonsillectomy. But this came about almost by accident—the kind of accident, as Pasteur said of vaccination, that 'favours prepared minds'. Previously, following tonsillectomy under local anaesthesia, the patient usually complained of sore throat and inability to eat or drink for several days. Since acupuncture was noted to be effective in relieving sore throat and pharyngitis the question arose as to why the procedure should not be used for post-operative sore throat. It proved highly successful and acupuncture was later used as anaesthesia for the tonsillectomy itself with even greater success.

The success of acupuncture anaesthesia in experiments on 660 medical personnel and other volunteers, led to 40,000 other trial cases over the next few years. This in turn led psychiatrists to experiment with possible new methods of treatment for psychiatric diseases, on the theory that it should be possible to transmit electricity through the sensory nerves to the higher centres of the brain without adversely affecting the motor cortex, as happens in electric shock treatment.

Traditionally, psychiatric treatment aimed at inhibiting the activities of the cerebrum, the physiological as well as the pathological symptoms being suppressed. When acupuncture—using electrical stimulation—was tried it appeared to suppress only the pathological activities. It did not influence the physiological activities of the cerebrum at all. In the Shanghai Psychiatric Hospital more than 1200 patients were treated and approximately 73 per cent showed good to fair response.[3]

One patient in a catatonic stupor, lay completely motionless in bed, did not eat, drink or utter a word. His dependence on others was total. Previously, the only treatment for this condition had been electric shock therapy, but the relapse rate was always high. After electrical stimulation of his acupuncture points a few times the patient gradually recovered, and not only ate and drank normally but also talked rationally.

The indications from this and the other cases listed above were that in certain ways the application of electro-acupuncture through the trigeminal nerve was analogous to the evolution of external to internal pacemaker for heart stimulation. In order to overcome the impedance of the skin and chest wall, the external pacemaker needs a current of 60 to 70 volts and causes annoying stimulation of many somatic muscles. The internal pacemaker, with the tip of the electrode in the right ventricular cavity, needs a current of only one millivolt and does not stimulate any surrounding structure.[3]

The first successful use of acupuncture anaesthesia followed tonsillectomy surgery. Similarly, direct stimulation of the trigeminal nerve was conceived about the same time, following appendicitis surgery. The four points used were located in the distribution of the first and second branches of the trigeminal nerve, and were stimulated with great success.[4]

Experiments were conducted on animals as well as humans. Sensitive electronic instruments were attached to the brain, and the electric activity of the brain recorded. Stimulation of the trigeminal nerve elicited the strongest and widest distribution of the electric waves. On the other hand, stimulation of other cranial nerves induced much weaker electric waves of much smaller distribution.

[3] *Liberation Daily News*, 22 January 1972. [4] *Liberation Daily News*, 5 January 1972.

As the effects of acupuncture had been demonstrated to mediate through the nervous system, Chinese doctors experimented by ignoring acupuncture points and stimulating the areas rich in nerve endings, even the peripheral nerves—with equally satisfactory results. It was further discovered that the closer the stimulus was applied to the site of operation, the better the anaesthetic effect. The results after manual stimulation by twirling the needle and after electrical stimulation were compared, and it was found that the anaesthetic effect was almost the same.

The ear and external ear canal is a highly innervated area, supplied by fibres of the trigeminal, facial and vagus nerves of the cranial nerve system, and the greater and lesser occipital nerves of the cervical spinal nerve system. The nerve endings are closely interwoven and superimposed on each other. Since these nerves have a very wide distribution, stimulation of the branches in the ear has an analgesic effect on practically all parts of the body.

The Chinese claim that they can treat any part of the body through the ear alone, and their 1974 Ear Chart shows some 70 'acupuncture points'. It is interesting to note that the *cavum conchae* of the ear contains their lung, heart and liver 'points', and also a recently discovered area called 'muscle relaxing point'. The significance of this juxtaposition will be explained later.

Electro-analgesia in the West

In the West, success with electro-analgesia was first reported in 1967, on stimulation of peripheral nerves. Drs P. D. Wall and W. H. Sweet reported successful treatment of eight patients with severe cutaneous pain by stimulation of their peripheral nerves.[5] The following year Drs W. A. Sweet and J. G. Wespic reported success in some of their eighteen patients with chronic intermittent peripheral stimulation.[6] Then in 1974 Drs P. W. Nathan and P. D. Wall described treating 30 patients suffering from severe post-herpetic neuralgia with prolonged self-administered electric

5 'Temporary Abolition of Pain in Man', *Science*, 155, pp. 108-109.
6 'Treatment of Chronic Pain by Stimulation of Fibres of Primary Afferent Neurons', *Trans-America Neural Association*, 93, pp. 103-7.

stimulation from a portable apparatus. The results were good in eleven cases. In eight of these the course of the neuralgia was improved, and two were cured.[7]

The two Western acupuncture authorities mentioned earlier, Dr Felix Mann and Dr Louis Moss, had both emphasized the important part played by the nervous system in acupunctural stimulation. Dr Felix Mann had declared:

'I think the neurophysiological theory to explain the mechanism of acupuncture, which I have developed over the past years . . . will soon be recognized as the basis for the scientific investigation and further development of acupuncture . . .'

And Dr Louis Moss had said:

'Chinese acupuncturists are taught that all illnesses stem from an imbalance of the flow of energy and that these can be cured and relieved by stimulation of the affected meridians at certain points of acupuncture. Without doubt the autonomic nervous system plays an important role.'[8]

These conclusions by Western doctors and scientists were being confirmed by different groups of Chinese doctors and scientists working in separate fields. A report from the Kuang-si Medical College Acupuncture Anaesthesia Group[9] concluded that the reticular formation played an important role. Some of the evidence was summarized as follows:

1. the effectiveness of acupuncture anaesthesia depended to a certain degree on the mental state of the patient, being more effective if the patient was calm, cooperative and confident, and less effective if the patient was agitated and fearful.
2. the effectiveness of acupuncture anaesthesia varied from patient to patient.
3. acupuncture could generate many regulatory effects on bodily functions such as the blood pressure, pulse, respiration and gastrointestinal motility.

7 'Treatment of Post-Herpetic Neuralgia by Prolonged Electric Stimulation', *British Medical Journal*, 1974, 3, pp. 645-647.
8 *Acupuncture and You.*
9 'Activities of the Recticular Formation of the Brain Stem under Acupuncture Anaesthesia', *Kuang Ming Daily News*, 31 January 1972.

In his book, *The Puzzle of Pain*,[10] Ronald Melzack describes the inhibitory effect that the central tegmental tract has on input.

'The inhibitory influence may help to explain an exciting recent discovery. Reynolds (1969, 1970) has observed that electrical stimulation in the region of the central grey and central tegmental tract produces a marked analgesia in rats, so that they fail to respond to pinch, burn, even major abdominal surgery . . . More recently, Mayer, Walfle, Akil, Carder and Liebeskin (1971) observed the same phenomenon, and found, moreover, that there is some somatotopic organisation within the system, so that stimulation at a given site produces analgesia of only selected positions of the body, such as the lower half, or one quadrant. They found, furthermore, that the electrical stimulation of these areas appears 'pleasurable' to the animals—they actively seek it out by pressing a lever to stimulate themselves. These observations . . . have great theoretical significance since they suggest the presence of a system that exerts a tonic, widespread inhibitory influence on transmission through the somatosensory projection system . . .'

Neural effects and chemical changes

According to recent neurophysiological studies two of the most prominent activities of the reticular formation is the downstream influence upon the spinal cord and the peripheral motor system, and the upstream influence upon the cerebral cortex. The reticular formation also exercises regulatory control over many visceral and vascular activities. Melzack also points out:

'There is now more direct evidence of prolonged changes in spinal cord activity. Spencer and April (1970) have shown that a seven-minute period of intense high-frequency "tetanic" electrical stimulation of sensory fibres produces a change—post tetanic potentiation—in a simple spinal cord reflex for more than ten minutes after stimulation is stopped. Twenty minutes stimula-

10 Penguin Education, 1973.

tion produces potentiation for more than two hours. Potentiation lasting an hour or more occurs even with stimulus frequencies as low as one hundred pulses per second for twenty to thirty minutes . . . There is also evidence of prolonged activity in brain tissue. Melzack, Konrad and Dubrovsky (1968, 1969) have observed that brief (ten to twenty seconds) stimulation of the skin or sciatic nerve in moderately anaesthetised cats produces marked, prolonged changes in the tonic, spontaneous activity at several synaptic levels of the skin sensory system, the brainstem reticular formation, and other discrete brain areas . . .'

The Kuang-si Medical College Group carried out 52 experiments on normal animals, and anaesthetic effects of various degrees were obtained 43 times, making the rate of effectiveness some 82 per cent. The average induction time was 11 minutes 30 seconds. The animals were then injected with many kinds of medicine which were known to have an effect on the central nervous system—sedatives, hypnotics, analgesics, anaesthetics, central stimulants, anti-depressants, tranquillisers, psychotherapeutic agents, and autonomic drugs such as cholinergic and cholinergic-blocking agents, and adrenergic and adrenergic-blocking agents. The anaesthetic effect of acupuncture was compared before and after the administration of these drugs and it was found that some increased the effectiveness of acupuncture anaesthesia, whereas others invariably reduced it.

Another group, the Research Group of Acupuncture Anaesthesia of the Peking Medical College, conducted and filmed a series of experiments with rabbits. I saw this film in Hong Kong.[11] They studied the parts played by various brain chemicals in acupuncture analgesia and especially the effects of substances that were known to be involved in the transmission of nerve impulses and thus were probably concerned in the sensations of pain and analgesia.

In the film two rabbits had their circulations linked, but only one received acupuncture to induce analgesia; yet the pain

[11] Later published in *Scientia Sinica*, February 1974.

threshold was raised significantly in *both* animals. In another experiment the cerebro-spinal fluid from one acupunctured rabbit was transferred to a non-acupunctured rabbit with considerable rise in the pain threshold of the second rabbit, but not as marked as in the first rabbit.

In the case of the rabbits, acupuncture by finger pressure was used rather than the widely-known needles, since too much local tissue damage occurred when needles were used. Some Chinese claim that from the historical point of view finger acupuncture was probably the first method used, and it has come increasingly into favour. This was to have considerable significance in my later development of electrodes in stimulation.

Since previous reports had suggested that monoamines in the brain are especially important in analgesia the Chinese scientists depleted the test rabbits of monoamines by administering the drug reserpine to block the effect of morphine as an analgesic. Surprisingly, it enhanced the effects of acupuncture. When the monoamines dopamine and 5-hydroxytryptamine were restored to the brain artificially, the effects of acupuncture analgesia returned to normal, and morphine was again effective.

Conversely, when they similarly tested the effects of the neurotransmitter substance acetylcholine, they found that it played an important part in acupuncture analgesia. When acetylcholine action was blocked by atropine the effect of acupuncture was very much weakened. Morphine analgesia was not affected by interference with acetylcholine by intraventricular injection of atropine.

Later reports in the West confirmed the importance of these investigations. The London *Times* Science Report declared:

'As well as providing valuable and interesting evidence that the mechanism of acupuncture analgesia is different from that mediated by morphine the parallel experiments run with morphine show that the methods of investigation and measurement that the authors are using are valid and that the conclusions they draw are to be considered seriously. There seems little doubt that acupuncture produces changes that result in the blocking of pain impulses in the brain . . .[12]

Researches in the West have also demonstrated that electrical stimulation of certain areas in the brain of rats and cats makes animals 'become totally unresponsive to pain while retaining a normal ability to respond to other stimuli' and that the analgesic effect can outlast the stimulation by several hours. They have also demonstrated that stimulation-produced analgesia is facilitated by serotinin and dopamine and antagonized by norepinephrine.[13]

Electro-anaesthesia

Electro-anaesthesia is not new, or even introduced from China. Research for an alternative to chemical anaesthesia began in 1902 at the Hospital Necker in Paris where Professor François Leduc discovered that certain high frequency electric currents had an anaesthetising effect.

By 1966 (when the first international symposium on electro-anaesthesia and electro-sleep was held in Europe) Professor Aimé Limoge, at the faculty of dental surgery at the University of Paris, had developed his research to the point of designing a generator which he claimed would produce a high frequency current that would keep a patient anaesthetised for as long as necessary. Unlike electro-convulsive therapy, where the current is of short duration and the patient remains unconscious for some time afterward, in electrical anaesthesia the patient can have a long period of current and can awake immediately.

The first operation using electro-anaesthesia was successfully performed at Hospital Necker in 1972, and within four months the French Academy of Medicine authorized the use of the technique. Since then the Necker medical team have performed over 400 operations using electro-anaesthesia. Lengthy operations, such as arterial grafting, kidney transplantation and other urological and intestinal procedures, are common. Two other

12 *The Times*, 28 March 1974.

13 D. J. Mayer, 'Pain Inhibition by Electrical Brain Stimulation: Comparison to Morphine', *Neurosciences Research Progress Bulletin*, Vol. 13, No. 1, 1975, pp. 94-100.

hospitals have now introduced electro-anaesthesia and are using it for major heart surgery. The longest operation to date at the Necker Hospital has been for ten-and-a-half hours.

According to a recent report in *World Medicine* (15 January 1975):

'. . . The success of the anaesthesia depends on the choice of starter drug, the position of the electrodes and the type of current used . . . The exact location of the electrodes is crucial and it took Professor Limoge two years to find the optimum positions: the cathode between the eyebrows and the two anodes, one behind each mastoid. Professor Limoge's electric generator produces a unidirectional current of 100KHz which is modified in a rectangular signal 3msec long with a frequency of 77Hz. There is a 10 msec pause between each signal and the current varies between 5 and 15 mA with a voltage of 10–25 volts. This steady current is sufficient to sustain anaesthesia for as long as is necessary and the patient regains consciousness as soon as the electrodes are disconnected . . . Because of rapid recovery the patient does not have the usual wooziness felt on awakening from conventional anaesthesia.'

An interesting point is that electro-anaesthesia seems to produce a lingering post-operative analgesic effect which lasts between six and forty-eight hours. Professor Limoge reckons that in the immediate post-operative days patients receive only one-thirtieth the analgesics and soporifics they need after conventional anaesthesia. It is also worth noting that there were abscesses in only 3 per cent of 180 cases anaesthetised by cerebral electro-therapy whereas in the same hospital in 100 random cases anaesthetised by conventional anaesthesia, there were abscesses in 17 per cent.[14]

Electro-sleep

In 1966 twenty years had passed since a new method of neurotropic therapy, namely electro-sleep, was evolved by Soviet scientists. Its introduction was preceded by numerous physio-

14 *Fourth International Symposium on Electrosleep and Electroanaesthesia*, Paris, 1975.

logical studies both in the USSR and elsewhere of the effects of electric current on the animal and human brain and investigations of phenomena of local and general electro-anaesthesia.

Sleep therapy, based on Pavlov's concept of sleep as protective inhibition, was widely acclaimed as an important addition to therapeutic measures, comparing favourably with the disadvantages associated with drug-induced sleep. However, in spite of the acceptance of electro-sleep as a therapeutic method both in the USSR and Europe, its widespread successes in clinical practice, and extensive theoretical and experimental research (over 450 publications), so far no uniformity of viewpoints had emerged—either on the mechanism of induction of electro-sleep or on the mechanism of its therapeutic effect.

One example of treatment was given by a Russian doctor, G. V. Sergeev of the Institute of Internal Medicine, USSR Academy of Medical Sciences, Moscow, in a paper entitled 'The Use of Electro-sleep in Clinical Medicine':

'Electro-sleep, as a factor exerting a neurotropic action on the central nervous system, is used in clinical medicine for the treatment of various diseases with underlying disturbances of the cortical regulation of somatic function . . .'

The author's technique: 'rectangular pulse, constant polarity, duration of pulse 0.2-0.3 msec, current intensity 15-20 mA expressing the amplitude value of the pulse at a frequency of 80-100 pulses per sec., daily sessions lasting from 30 minutes to 2 hours, course of treatment of up to 20-25 sessions . . .'

F. M. Wageneder, of the University Surgical Clinic, Graz, Austria, in a paper, 'Report on Eight years Experience in the Area of Electro-sleep Therapy', stated that the designation 'electro-sleep therapy' was misleading, in that sometimes patients who failed to sleep during treatments were therapeutic successes. He proposed 'cerebral electro-therapy' as a more appropriate term, since it expressed more accurately the real nature of the treatment.

The indications for cerebral electro-therapy, he suggested from his experience, might be classified under the general heading of 'all disorders, with psycho-autonomic manifestations'.

Although electro-anaesthesia and electro-sleep were outside my immediate field of research, the intensive research being conducted by specialists—particularly in Russia and Europe—in the area of parameters of current I found to be of considerable significance in my own researches.

Chapter Three

Development of Treatment

Various forms of stimulation have been used by the Chinese in addition to the 'needle' and 'finger' acupuncture. Injection acupuncture entails the injection of sterile water, saline, morphine, etc. into acupuncture points. 'Thread acupuncture' passes catgut threaded to a surgical needle from one acupuncture point to another. 'Pressure acupuncture' consists of the application of pressure on the skin over the acupuncture points.

Stimulation is achieved either manually through a push-pull and rotary movement or, in the case of electro-acupuncture, by a regulatory current. Manual stimulation is carried out for 10 to 15 minutes and the needle either removed or left in place, according to choice. Then after an interval the procedure is repeated.

Electro-acupuncture eliminated the need repeatedly to twirl the needles, and gained widespread use in acupuncture anaesthesia because it produced continued stimulation over longer periods of time with much less effort on the part of the operator. Also, the strength of stimulation could be adjusted according to the needs of the patient, and a stronger stimulation could be achieved than with manual stimulation.

A number of electro-acupuncture stimulators were developed, but after wide experience, three models became most popular in China—the BT-701, the G6805, and the 6.26.

Dr Wen, Dr Cheung and I started with the 6.26 model, which had a wide bipolar spike wave form, AC current, pulse width 0.6 msec and a frequency up to 111 Hz or cycles per second (cps).[1]

[1] Later, on arrival in England, I had this machine tested. See Appendix I.

Experimentation in Hong Kong

Over a period of three months we treated 40 cases of drug addiction in the Tung Wah Group of Hospitals, Hong Kong.[2] Thirty of these patients were opium addicts and the other 10, heroin addicts. Of these 40 cases, six came voluntarily for treatment of drug addiction; the remainder for a variety of conditions.[3] The average amount of drug-taking varied considerably, but the official average daily drug intake in Hong Kong is given as HK$8.6 and at that time this bought 900 milligrammes of 40-60 per cent heroin mixed with 60-40 per cent barbitone.

We modified the standard techniques for inducing analgesia through electro-acupuncture by using the ears only. In acupuncture terminology we used the 'lung' point in the middle of the concha and here we inserted needles on each side between the skin and the cartilage for a depth of ½cm, then connected the needles by crocodile clips and leads to the stimulator. The intensity was increased until the patient felt the flow of current in the ear as a slight tingling and this was retained for an average of 30-40 minutes per treatment, with two or three treatments a day for three to five days during the acute withdrawal stage, followed by one treatment for the subsequent four or five days.

Uniform results were obtained about 10 to 15 minutes after stimulation began. The patients' eyes, nose and mouth became dry; the aching, shivering and abdominal pain decreased; breathing became regular and they felt warm and relaxed.

Drs Wen and Cheung have reported their results in *The Asian Journal of Medicine*:

'Of the 40 cases, 39 were discharged and are free of drug addiction (one was transferred to another hospital for surgery of tumour of the bladder). These patients have gained weight and said that they have since had no urge to take the drug. Twenty-two of these cases had their urine sent for investigation, to see if it was positive for the drugs. The report showed one doubtful

2 Dr H. L. Wen and Dr S. Y. C. Cheung, 'Treatment of Drug Addiction by Acupuncture and Electrical Stimulation', *The Asian Journal of Medicine*, Vol. 9, April 1973.

3 See Appendix II for Table provided by Dr Wen.

case, and one positive case . . . The "doubtful" result related to a case of concussion, who had been put on Luminal for post-concussional syndrome. The one positive case was suffering from tumour of the bladder, which necessitated injections of narcotic to stop his pain. The 20 cases which showed negative urine tests are free of the drug and so far have no urge for it either . . . Up to the present eight cases have come back to have one or two repetitions of the treatment . . . Each of them was given the treatment as an out-patient, and so far they have had no recurrence of the symptoms . . .'

By the time I left Hong Kong in July 1973, over 100 cases of heroin and opium addiction had been treated, with similar results.

The successful treatment of these patients, with others I was treating privately in Hong Kong, opened up new fields of possible curative potential in hitherto intractable conditions. And in seeking to discover the possible mechanisms of cure—both from sources inside China and the West—I became aware that parallel, but isolated, investigations into the significance of electrical stimulation were taking place which together might provide a unique historical contribution.

Official discouragement in Hong Kong

Unfortunately, Hong Kong, although in so many ways the ideal place to conduct such research—adjacent to China, a rich Colony, with a huge drug problem and good hospitals—was also the least likely place to help, because of the sensitive, almost paranoid, official attitude towards the drug problem. Out of a four million population, the officially admitted number of drug addicts was given as 100,000, although this figure has been ridiculed by informed researchers, who point out that it was only acquired as a guess from dubious statistics and that a more likely figure is 250,000. Certainly, from my own experience during nine years in a totally Chinese hospital, we calculated that we had a regular 10-15 per cent of addicted patients in our general wards. But even the officially admitted 100,000 constitutes, proportionately, the highest drug addiction rate in the world.

However, because of the financial, social and political factors involved, the authorities were more concerned with concealing the scale of the problem than with finding a possible medical solution. Consequently, pressure was applied to Drs Wen, Cheung and myself to put a stop to all experimenting with acupuncture anaesthesia. It could not be stopped legally because acupuncture, as traditional Chinese medicine, was allowed to be practised in Hong Kong by law. But in addition to strongly-worded circulars issued by the official medical authorities threatening severe consequences, there were warnings against public lectures (Dr Wen had given one to a packed audience of doctors), pressure through the hospital (we were conducting our research in addition to our own surgical responsibilities), and official denials to the local and international press that anything medically significant in the area of drug addiction cure had happened.

Successful treatment of status asthmaticus

In the meantime another of our colleagues in the Tung Wah Group of Hospitals, Dr K. Chau, my physician counterpart, had been experimenting by using the same methods in the treatment of status asthmaticus. He had found that it produced better results than any achieved by conventional therapy. The investigations were conducted from December 1972—March 1973.

During this period, all 30 cases of bronchial asthma under the care of the Medical Unit of the Tung Wah Hospital were offered acupuncture and electro-stimulation therapy. Of the patients under observation, six had particularly severe bronchial asthma. They all had had recurrent attacks of severe status asthmaticus, a history of repeated hospital admissions for asthma within the preceding 12 months, and symptoms that interfered with work and sleep. In all six patients the asthmatic attacks were worse in winter. Four had associated emphysema. Three of them had been under the care of the Unit for more than three consecutive years prior to the investigations and had previously received short-term cortico-steroid therapy during approximately half of their hospital admission because of poor response to other treatments. The other three patients had been treated previously in other hospitals, and had come into the Unit as emergency cases with severe asthmatic attacks. One of them had continuous asthma for two months before being admitted.[4]

Dr Chau has also reported his findings in *The Asian Journal of Medicine*:[5]

'All patients showed significant objective response to acupuncture and electro-stimulation therapy. Table 2 shows the value of pulmonary-function tests before and at half hour after therapy for mild to moderately severe asthmatic attacks in the six patients studied. All patients showed significant improvement in FEVI, FVC and PEFR after treatment. The response was least in the patient who had severe emphysema (Case 3). Fig 1 shows the successive measurements of PEFR taken every five minutes in one patient (Case 1) during two separate asthmatic attacks. Significant improvement of PEFR appeared five minutes after commencement of acupuncture and electro-stimulation in a mild attack and in 10 minutes in a moderate attack.

'The result of the present study indicates that in the patients studied, acupuncture and electro-stimulation therapy is superior to conventional therapy in the management of severe bronchial asthma and status asthmaticus. It is superior in the aspects of potency of action, duration of effect, minimum of side effects, and absence of resistance to therapy. In the present study, it has been utilised successfully in the treatment of acute asthmatic attacks including status asthmaticus, in regular follow-up treatment as out-patients after discharge and in one patient it has successfully replaced all other forms of therapy for bronchial asthma for a period of one month . . .'

Dr Chau had been led to experiment with status asthmaticus because of three indications:

1. the treatment of asthma by Chinese acupuncturists used sites in the external ear;

[4] See Appendix III for Tables.

[5] Dr H. L. Wen and Dr K. Chau, 'Status Asthmaticus Treated by Acupuncture and Electro-Stimulation', *The Asian Journal of Medicine*, Vol. 9, June 1973, pp. 191ff.

2. in asthmatic attacks, the bronchial spasm is caused by the activity of the para-sympathetic nervous system, stimulated through the vagus nerve;
3. the external ear canal and concha are richly endowed with the peripheral branches of the facial, glosso-pharyngeal and vagus nerves, all associated with the para-sympathetic nervous system.

Dr Wen, placed under considerable restraint by the officials in Hong Kong, continued his private investigations into acupuncture anaesthesia and its applications to brain operations. In China, from December 1965 to August 1972, a total of 482 cases of craniotomy were performed under acupuncture anaesthesia at the Peking Hsuan Wu Hospital.[6] And from November 1965 to July 1972 the results of 619 cases of neuro-surgery under acupuncture were analysed by the Shanghai First Medical College[7] which claimed an over-all success rate of 96.3 per cent in the series. Later Dr Wen presented the results of 20 cases of his own, with only two failures.[8]

Importance of the electrical factor in stimulation

I became increasingly convinced that it was the electrical stimulation of the nerve pathways, rather than the acupuncture points, that was the important factor. When I varied the frequencies and wave-forms I found them in some cases to be inadequate. For example, the Chinese addicts would often describe a treatment of 111 cps as being 'like HK$5 (300 mgms) of heroin'. But when an English addict came off his Methadone in 4 days of therapy (with no other drugs given), yet found that his craving for the stimulant I.V. Ritalin (Methyl Phenictate Hydrochlor.) was undiminished, I deduced that a much higher frequency might control his craving. This meant using a different machine from any of the machines available from China. Later, after I had

6 'Acupuncture Anaesthesia in Neurosurgery', *Chinese Medical Journal*, 53(2): 67, 1973.
7 'Observations on Analgesic Effect of Needling Chuanliao Point in Surgery', *Chinese Medical Journal*, 53(2): 21, 1973.
8 Dr H. L. Wen, 'Acupuncture Anaesthesia for Neurosurgery', *The Asian Journal of Medicine*, Vol. 10, May 1974.

developed a machine to my own specifications, I found this deduction proved when I used 2000 cps to relieve the cravings of I.V. Ritalin. (Unexpectedly, one alcoholic and two nicotine addicts have also responded better to this frequency than to any other, whereas the majority of addicts to alcohol, heroin, methadone and nicotine responded to lower frequencies.)

On returning to London for further research I applied for a grant to the Medical Research Council. They were interested and sympathetic, but refused my application. However, they officially encouraged me to pursue my investigations in my spare time. Fortunately, because of the personal interest and co-operation of several friends and patients I was able to carry on with my research.

Andrew Grima, a well-known London jeweller, worked with me for several months to provide a suitable ear-clip incorporating a needle so tiny that it caused no pain. I had found that Europeans could not tolerate the pain of the Chinese needles in their ears. David Shackman, of Shackman Instruments Ltd., put all his firm's facilities at my disposal, and his managing director, Geoff Bennett, provided endless patience and advice as well as considerable expertise, to produce a suitable stimulator (the only stimulators available in Britain were imported from America and after trial were proved inadequate for my purpose).

Finally, because of the successful treatment of internationally famous music personalities, Robert Stigwood of the Robert Stigwood Organisation provided me with the necessary grant to pursue my researches for two years. But it took a full year before I was given official permission to carry out a pilot project in one of the National Health Service Clinics, unpaid, and also with no money supplied for the machines which I had developed and which I now had to provide to treat the registered addicts. I never succeeded in getting permission from the Department of Health and Social Security to conduct a similar project with alcoholics, despite the eagerness of local staff to participate.

The Shackman-Patterson machine which we developed[9]

had a variety of wave-forms, pulse widths from 0.1 to 1.5 msec and frequencies varying from 5 to 2000 cps. This transistorized machine included both the standard square or rectangular wave form used in neuro-electric treatment[10] and in intra-cranial implantations[11] and the spike wave form used by the Chinese, who presumably—although not stated in any publication available outside China—have some special reason for using this particular wave form. The machine could also insert a modulation of 50 KHz. (I only later discovered that French researchers were inserting a 100 KHz modulated signal in their electro-anaesthesia machine.)

In the first six months of research (November 1973 to June 1974) my tentative conclusions were that the twirling of the acupuncture needle was producing a mild electrical current and thereby was altering the electrical phenomena inherent in every neurone. Also from the clinical evidence emerging, there were indications that there might be regeneration of neurones or, at least, a reconditioning of some brain circuits, such as the reticular formation. Consequently, I arranged an additional programme of research into the electrical phenomena associated with acupunctural stimulation, in collaboration with Dr Alfred C. C. Tseung, BSc, PhD, CEng, FRCIS, FTCeram, PIM, Minst. F, Reader in the Department of Chemistry of the City University, London, under the general heading of 'Acupuncture Analgesia and its Possible Mechanisms of Action' and 'The Possible Interpretation of Electro-Acupuncture Based on Electrochemical Ideas'. To date, evidence is emerging that may help to explain the clinical effects of electrochemical stimulation, for example, that different intensities of electric current can rapidly reduce alcohol either to the toxic aldehydes or to the non-toxic CO_2 and water.

9 See Appendix IV for photographs, diagrams and specifications.

10 Schuy, Gonser, Mageneder and Mansoner, Anaesthetic Department Surgical Clinic, University of Graz, Austria, *First International Symposium*, 1966: 1, 82, et al.

11 Dr Irving S. Cooper, MD, 'Chronic Stimulation of Cerebellar Cortex in the Human', *Neural Organisation*, 1973, 373.

Chapter Four
Associated Medical/Electronic Treatments

How the process of addiction works has long been a mystery, and without this knowledge it has not been possible to develop a successful treatment of addiction. But recently several independent medical researchers have come up with findings that have improved the hitherto pessimistic situation.

Addiction and electrical stimulation

Although it was the Chinese acupuncture anaesthetic techniques which caught the imagination of the scientific West following President Nixon's visit, the possibilities of electrical stimulation had been recognized in the West for some time.

A series of 'Skinner box' experiments investigating causes of drug dependence in rats—having a stimulating electrode permanently implanted in the medial forebrain bundle of the brain and wired so that this bundle of neurones was shocked when the rat pressed a lever—have indicated noradrenaline as the main mediator of reward. One such experiment used 6-hydroxydopamine, which depresses catecholamine biosynthesis and destroys nerve terminals producing a catecholamine. When 6-hydroxydopamine was injected into the cisterna magna of the brain of six rats prepared for electrical self-stimulation, the rate at which the animals pressed the lever to obtain an electric shock in the medial forebrain bundle was roughly halved. A second injection virtually eliminated self-stimulation in five of the six rats. Yet another experiment which indicated that noradrenaline is the catecholamine that excites the cerebral reward system of the rat was done with disulfiram and diethyldithiocarbamate. These drugs blocked the conversion of dopamine to noradrenaline. The inhibited self-stimulation of the animals was restored by injecting noradrenaline into a cerebral ventricle. Thus, at this stage, the proposition seems well-founded that drugs of dependence induced euphoria by enhancing catecholaminergic mechanisms in the brain. The important question arose whether electrical stimulation did the same.

Describing the significance of the 'Skinner box' experiments, H. O. J. Collier, BA, PhD, ScD, FJ Biol said:[1]

'In animals whose psychic processes are observable through their behaviour we may speak of "behavioural dependence" which may include psychic and physical components . . . An animal is usually prepared in dependence studies with an intravenous cannula connected to an infusion pump, which is activated by a lever in the wall of the cage. By pressing the lever the animal can self-inject drugs . . . If the rat is offered a strong instead of a weak solution of heroin the pattern of its lever-pressing will be different. It will learn to press the lever more and more often.

'An analogy can be drawn between self-injection of a rewarding drug and the behaviour seen when an animal is prepared so that it can stimulate electrically a certain point in its own brain. To obtain the latter behaviour, a stimulating electrode is implanted in the medial forebrain bundle of the brain. The electrode is wired so that this bundle of neurones is shocked when the rat presses a lever in the wall of the Skinner box. In this situation a rat will usually stimulate its brain several thousand times an hour . . .

'In the most general terms a multiplication induced by the drug of dependence, of some kind of receptor on enzyme, carrier, neurone, or storage site that handles, or reacts to, an active endogenous substance mediating or modulating neuronal responses, appears to be nearest to explaining dependence . . .'

Then in March 1973, Dr Solomon Snyder and researcher Candace Pert of the Johns Hopkins University School of Medicine reported in the US journal *Science* that they had succeeded in

1 'The Experimental Analysis of Drug Dependence', *ICI*, September 1972.

locating the receptor sites that attract opiates. The area of the brain where the researchers found the heaviest concentration of opiate receptors is the corpus striatum, which seems to play a part in integrating motor activity and perceptual information. The receptors occurred much less frequently in the cerebral cortex, which regulates higher intellectual functions, and the brain stem which controls sleeping and wakefulness. Snyder concluded that the ideal opiate antagonist should be potent, long-lasting, non-addictive, orally administered and free from side effect. Such a substance when given over a period of time to an ex-addict would, he hoped, decondition his heroin-seeking behaviour and possibly result in psychological changes as well.

Epilepsy and stimulation

Electro-physiology began in the middle of the eighteenth century with some very mild experiments. Later on, awareness developed that not only was all living tissue sensitive to electric currents but that tissue itself generated small voltages, which changed considerably when it was injured or became active. In 1875 an English physician found that the brain also produced such currents.

From these early investigations there emerged the theory of four basic rhythmic patterns which were named alpha, beta, delta and theta. Delta rhythms are the slowest, running between 1 and 3 cycles per second, and are most prominent in deep sleep. Theta rhythms are those with a frequency of 4 to 7 cycles per second, which seemed to be connected with mood. From 8 to 12 cycles are the rhythms which occur most often in relaxed meditation. And beta rhythms, between 13 and 22 cycles per second, seemed to be confined to the frontal area of the brain, where complex mental processes take place.

In 1946 Dr W. Grey Walter, now one of Britain's leading neuro-physiologists, decided to try imposing new patterns of the existing brain rhythms through the senses. He began by flashing a light at regular intervals into the subject's eyes and found that this flicker produced new, strange patterns on the graphs. At certain frequencies the flicker also produced violent reactions in the subject, who was suddenly seized by what seemed to be an epileptic fit.[2]

Grey Walter also noted the similarity of a natural epileptic seizure and one induced by electric shock therapy. He then turned his investigations to normal, resting brain waves of known epileptics and found that their brain rhythms were grouped in certain frequencies. In order to keep the flicker and the brain in time, a feedback system in automatic control was adopted in the form of a trigger-circuit, the flash being fired by the brain rhythms themselves at any chosen time relation with any rhythmic component of the spontaneous or evoked activity. With this instrument the effects of flicker were found to be even more drastic than when the stimulus was fixed by an operator, in that in more than 50 per cent of young normal adult subjects the first exposure to feedback flicker evoked transient paroxysmal discharges of the type seen so often in epileptics.

'It was as if certain major chords constantly appeared against the trills and arpeggios of the normal activity,' Grey Walter reported. This harmonic grouping suggested to him that all that was necessary to get the rhythms to synchronize in a tremendous explosion was an outside co-ordinator, a conductor who could bring the separate chords together, in a simultaneous grand convulsion. A flicker in the alpha-rhythm range, between 8 and 12 cycles a second, acted in just this way on epileptics, provoking them into a seizure at any time. This technique has now become a valuable clinical aid in the diagnosis of epilepsy.

The cerebellum and stimulation

About the same time (1950) Dr Irving Cooper—later to be known as 'the father of cryogenic surgery', but then a Fellow in Neuro-Surgery at the Mayo Foundation—read in a book by the Italian physiologist, Giuseppe Moruzzi, the remarkable observation that electrical stimulation of the anterior lobe of the cerebellum could

2 Dr W. Grey Walter, *The Living Brain*, Duckworth and Co., London.

produce either a decrease or an increase of decerebrate rigidity from the same point, depending upon the frequency of stimulation. He found that with frequencies of 10 cycles per second increase of decerebrate rigidity might be activated, while frequencies of 100 to 300 cps invariably produced a decrease. Also, the decrease of frequency of stimulation could be compensated for by increasing the duration of each stimulus. But a train of repetitive stimulation was always necessary in order to produce an inhibitory or facilitatory effect.

Twenty years later, in the winter of 1972, Dr Cooper began implanting electrodes on the cerebellum through a suboccipital craniotomy for cases of severe epilepsy and various spastic conditions. He came to the conclusion that cerebellar stimulation arrested both the clinical seizures and the concomitant ictal EEG discharge and that this suggested a possible cerebellar interference with electrical seizure discharge, as had already been demonstrated in animal experiments. Such a finding was in keeping with other observations of cerebellar function. For example, anterior cerebellar stimulation did not appear clinically to affect muscular tone in normal limbs but did lessen tone in spastic extremities. These observations led in turn to another hypothesis, that the cerebellum is a modulator which arises to the needs of the organism. He speculated, therefore, that chronic cerebellar stimulation leads to a build-up of chemical changes in neurotransmitter systems. If so, a possible eventual reconditioning or normalization of some abnormal brain functions mediated by chemical systems might take place during chronic stimulation of the cerebellar cortex. Over a period of about two years of such stimulation he found that there were no signs of undesirable motor, sensory, intellectual or emotional changes.[3]

Pain and stimulation

In 1967 Drs P. D. Wall and W. H. Sweet reported producing pain relief by stimulating the sensory nerves or roots supplying

[3] *The Cerebellum, Epilepsy, and Behaviour*, edited by I. S. Cooper, M. Riklan and R. S. Snider, Plenum Press, New York-London 1974, pp. 119-171.

painful areas in eight patients.[4] They explained their results by the 'gate theory'. The theory was that it has been demonstrated physiologically that all pain information travels to the spinal cord via small unmyelinated C fibres and that stimulation of the larger myelinated A fibres is never painful. Further, activity in the large A fibres inhibits, at the first spinal synapse, immediate subsequent activity from the smallest fibres considered essential to pain conduction. Melzack and Wall suggested that this mechanism normally acts as a 'gate' to balance pain and non-pain input.

Chronic, intractable pain in a sufferer usually implies that nearly all conservative medical and surgical procedures have been tried and have failed. At this point, the neuro-surgeon concerned is faced with the final decision—to destroy nervous system tissues in an attempt to sever the pathways of the pain stimulus to the brain. Yet even drastic surgical procedures may fail to reduce the pain.

But the alleviation of the pain by electrical stimulation—or to give its medical designation, 'electro-hypalgesia'—is based on the theory that stimulation (for example, of the dorsal column) interferes with and blocks the normal transmission of pain impulses to the brain. This represents an alternative mode of therapy for the neuro-surgeon, in place of the usual potentially addictive drugs, and/or surgery that can cause partial paralysis.

In 1968, Drs Sweet and Wespic[5] reported controlling 'causalgia-like pain' for 32 months with self-administered, transcutaneous electrical stimulation of the median nerve. They also treated other patients with different types of pain, e.g. atypical facial neuralgia (of 17 years' duration), by self-administered transcutaneous stimulation of the infra-orbital nerves.

These experiments and others led to the development by Medtronic Inc. of the Myelostat Dorsal Column Stimulator (DCS) and the Cutaneous Stimulation Device (CSD). The DCS system consists of an RF transmitter, a transmitting antenna and a stimulating lead. The battery-operated transmitter and antenna

[4] See p. 21.
[5] See p. 21.

are worn externally, while the receiver/lead is implanted. Power is supplied to the receiver by inductive coupling through the skin.

In operation the antenna is placed on the skin directly over the implanted receiver. The receiver shapes the RF signal into the appropriate wave-form and applies this pulse to the dorsal columns via an electrode implanted on the *dura mater*.

The transmitter case contains pulse-generating circuitry, a 9-volt battery, and the necessary controls to vary the stimulating voltage, frequency and pulse width.

However, Dr Ronald Melzack[6] claims that a much more effective method to selectively activate large fibres appears to be the direct electrical stimulation of sensory nerves. Two minutes of stimulation may abolish severe neuralgic pain for more than two hours, and there was significant relief of pain in six out of eight patients suffering from causalgic pain, including two who had not been helped by sympathectomy. Patients with cancer pain report that the pain is diminished during the period of stimulation but returns shortly after it is stopped, so they require almost continuous stimulation to produce significant relief.

Bio-feedback and brain rhythms

Then in 1970, an experiment conducted in Kansas, USA, confirmed a revolutionary new medical theory that had been gaining currency for the previous few years—that many bodily functions thought to be involuntary could, in fact, be controlled. The experiment, conducted by Dr Elmer Green, Director of the Menninger Foundation voluntary-controls project, was to attach EKG electrodes to the left hand and right ear of an Indian swami, while the swami stopped his own heart. Dr Green thought the swami meant he was going to give himself some kind of neurological shock; but the shock the swami was talking about was psychological.

Before the self-induced shock the swami's recorded heart-rate

6 *The Puzzle of Pain*, Penguin Education, pp. 197–8.

was smooth and even at 70 beats a minute. Then, suddenly, in the space of one beat, it jumped to nearly 300 beats per minute. The polygraph pens jerked up and down five times every second for a span of some 17 seconds.

Animal experiments had shown that it was possible to teach rats to control their hearts, but the swami's experiment was the start of a series of experiments to teach humans to learn this technique to cure muscle tension among other things. But also out of this and similar knowledge derived from the use of curare on rats was developed the technique of 'bio-feedback'.

All learning requires feedback. When learning to speak, it is essential to hear. A child who is hard of hearing speaks poorly, but give him a hearing aid and he may learn to speak like any normal child.

So by its very nature, bio-feedback implies the use of machines. A bio-feedback machine is any device that makes a person more aware of an internal bodily function than he normally would be and which the person uses in an attempt to control the function voluntarily. A stethoscope can be a bio-feedback machine if a person uses it to observe his own heart-beat, to learn what it feels like to have his heart-rate go up and down and to try to bring his heart under voluntary control.

Some of the claims of success for bio-feedback techniques are highly fanciful, but in a few areas the findings have been very interesting. Some of bio-feedback's greatest successes have been in relieving muscle tension. With special machinery that registers muscle activity with a tone, or electronic clicks, it is possible to learn to relax a muscle completely or to isolate a single motor neurone and learn to 'fire' it at will. Variations on this technique have been used to partially rehabilitate stroke victims, or to eliminate speech impediments in slow readers, or to cure facial tics.

A much-publicized technique has been the use of 'alpha-machines' which react to show that the user's brainwaves have entered the 'alpha state' of calm and relaxation. The alpha is a brain-wave with a frequency between about 8 and 13 cps. Brain waves are the constant undulations in electrical activity that occur in any living brain. These waves are picked up by sensitive electrodes on the scalp and transferred to an electro-encephalogram (EEG). Brain waves are a rough measure of mental activity; they are fastest during active attentive thought and slowest in deep sleep. Generally, stimulants such as caffeine and tobacco and amphetamines speed up the predominant brain waves, while alcohol, morphine, marijuana and decreased blood sugar tend to slow them down.

Post-operative stimulation

Yet another form of electrical stimulation has been used for the past three years by surgeons in Minneapolis, USA to help patients recover faster after major surgery. Two cardio-vascular surgeons, Drs A. A. Hymes and D. E. Raab, concluded from records kept on patients over a period of 2½ years who, were given 'light, tingling electrical stimulation treatment', that the electrical stimulators 'reduced their pain about 80 per cent, especially in preventing the fairly common problem of bowel paralysis after surgery'.

The 'Great Bordeaux Magnetic Machine'

Then in *The Sunday Times* of 7 January 1973, Lord Zuckerman, OM, FRS, declared:

'The French scientific world is profoundly divided over the value of an extraordinary machine—The Great Bordeaux Magnetic Machine—built in Bordeaux by a 60 year-old engineer called Antoine Priore. Using electro-magnetic radiation it appears to have inhibited the growth of cancerous tissue in rats, and cured sleeping sickness in mice . . .

'Professor Algrain is a highly distinguished physicist, and while he still declares himself unable to understand how Mr Priore's apparatus could possibly operate in the light of established laws of physics, he accepts that Professor Poutrizel's experiments do imply that somehow or other the radiations it produces did stimulate the defence mechanisms of the body . . .'

Cerebral palsy, spasticity and stimulation

A few months later, C. P. Snow, the well-known English writer and scientist, reviewing a book in the *New York Sunday Times* (12 August 1973)[7] told of the work of Dr Irving S. Cooper, Director of the Department of Neuro-surgery at St Barnabas Hospital for Chronic Diseases, one of the world's great centres of neuro-surgery. He described him as 'one of the most remarkable men alive', and 'professionally one of the great brain surgeons of the world'.

I have already mentioned meeting Dr Cooper in Hong Kong. In our subsequent correspondence and meetings Dr Cooper informed me that he had treated about 30 patients suffering from hypertonic states such as cerebral palsy, the sequelae of stroke, spastic hemiplegia due to head injury and amyo-trophic lateral sclerosis as well as intractable epilepsy, with dramatic success.[8]

The technique he used was to implant electrodes in the brain by surgery, and to control stimulation of the cerebellum by what Dr Cooper termed 'the prosthetic mobilization of the inhibitory potential of the cerebellar cortex'.

'The cerebellum is an inhibitory mechanism functioning somewhat as a rheostat,' Dr Cooper explained. 'It has a modulating function on the rest of the brain. The evidence for its function has built up over the years in animal experiments. What is new is the application of some of this knowledge to human disease.'

The 'Cooper Brain Pacemaker'

What Dr Cooper had devised to cure neural disorders was a 'Cooper Brain Pacemaker'. This consists of one or more plates of silicon-coated Dacron mesh, to which are attached four or eight pairs of platinum disc electrodes. The plates are placed on the patients' cerebellar cortex. At first the plates were placed on the anterior lobe alone, because most of the experimental

7 I. S. Cooper, MD., *The Victim Is Always the Same*, Harper and Row, New York, 1973.

8 During a series of lectures held in the National Institute for Nervous Diseases, Queen's Square, London, in November 1974 Dr Cooper described the follow-up of cerebellar stimulation in over 100 cases of spastic conditions and 15 cases of severe epilepsy, with equally impressive results. Eleven of the 15 epileptics remain totally seizure-free.

work concerned this area and it is the strongest inhibitor of seizure and motor activity. In certain patients, however, such as some with spasticity, the electrodes were placed only on the posterior lobe, which has strong connections with the motor cortex. Now, for better control all new patients receive stimulation of both lobes. Bipolar stimulation between four or more pairs of electrodes is produced simultaneously.

The electrode plates are connected with subcutaneous leads to a small radio frequency receiver that is implanted in the patient's chest before brain surgery begins. Electrode stimulation originates from a transmitter carried outside the body and occurs by trans-epidermal inductive coupling by means of an antenna that is taped on the patient's chest directly over the receiver. The transmitter itself is about the size of a cigarette package and can be carried in a pocket or purse.

All electrodes on each side are stimulated simultaneously; the current procedure is to stimulate the cerebellum continuously, but in two separate areas alternately. All units now have an automatic timer (the patients originally stimulated themselves). It is hoped that newer techniques will allow the apparatus to be completely buried in the patient.

Stimulation is carried out with rectangular pulses, of 1 msec width, with a rate of 7 to 200 cps, and an intensity of 0.5 to 14 volts. Generally speaking, epileptic patients receive stimulation at 10 cps and 10 volts, and spastic patients 200 cps and 10 volts, depending on the patient.

Dr Cooper believes it is unlikely that the natural course of cerebral palsy, or of the other diseases he is treating, will be changed by cerebellar stimulation. However, he does feel that '*prosthetic stimulation of the cerebellum may gradually recondition reflex functioning of some brain circuits*'.

He has observed behavioural changes in all his patients, even in the few who have had little or no physical improvement. All of his patients were independently evaluated by Dr Manuel Riklan, PhD, before and after surgery and in continued follow-up. Dr Riklan has summarized the observed changes as follows:

'1. reduction in anxiety, tension, and feelings of stress.
2. improvement in thinking and fluency of speech; increased alertness.
3. reduction in depression; increased feelings of optimism.
4. reduced feelings of anger and reduction in outbursts of aggression associated with seizures and between seizures; improved emotional control.'[9]

Possible structural change after stimulation

Earlier experiments in England—the significance of which would appear to have been overlooked until fairly recently—also demonstrated possible structural change after electrical stimulation. Dr L. S. Illis, Consultant Neurologist of the Wessex Neurological Centre, Southampton General Hospital, writing in *Nature* (5 July 1969) stated:

'Adult cats were anaesthetised with intraperitoneal Nembutal. A catheter in the left ventricle was connected by a two-way tap to normal saline and fixation material. The left fifth lumber root was exposed by enlarging the root foramen without disturbing the spinal cord dura mater, cardiac pacemaker electrodes were placed around the root and the root was stimulated with a 1 msec pulse, 300 cps, 2.5 volts . . .

'After stimulation of a single posterior root for 65 minutes, *changes were seen in the areas where mono-synaptic fibres are known to terminate* . . .' (my italics).[10]

In correspondence Dr Illis has since added: 'I was particularly interested in your comments about the possibility of electrical stimulation altering tissue growth. I thought you might be interested in some work showing the effect of repetitive stimulation on the central nervous system. Since publishing that paper I have come across two further reports of similar experiments, with similar results—re a structural change after stimulation.'

9 Symposium on 'The Cerebellum, Epilepsy and Behaviour,' held at St Barnabas Hospital, New York, US, August 1973.

10 'Enlargement of Spinal Cord Synapses after Repetitive Stimulations of a Single Posterior Root.'

Tissue regeneration and stimulation

One of the leading international authorities on the subject of tissue regeneration is Dr Robert Becker, MD, Professor of Orthopaedic Surgery at the Upstate Medical Centre, New York State and Medical Investigator at the Veterans' Administration Hospital in Syracuse, New York. Dr Becker had already succeeded in stimulating regeneration in laboratory animals and had begun to apply his technique to humans for fractured bones showing non-union.

Becker's work in tissue regeneration dated back to 1958 when he and his colleagues began experiments to determine whether electrical stimulation could trigger bone and other tissue growth in animals. Earlier research had already established that the chances of regeneration in a species depended on the proportion of nerve tissue in the area of regeneration. Becker pointed out that man, with roughly 70 per cent of his total nerve mass concentrated in his brain, cannot regenerate. But salamanders, with only half the mass of their nerve tissue in their brains and the remainder spread throughout their bodies, can grow new tails, legs and even heart tissue. Becker theorized that he could increase the regenerative powers of higher animals by somehow compensating for the relatively small proportion of nerve tissue in their extremities, by bolstering the electrical activity in the nerve network. After amputating limbs from 39 rats he planted electrodes in the amputation sites and applied current to stimulate cell changes. All but two of the animals responded with some limb growth; many regenerated amputated forelegs as far as the first joint.

More recently, in a paper presented at the Second International Symposium on Bioelectrochemistry in France, October 1973, entitled 'The Significance of Bio-electric Potentials', Becker expanded his theories to postulate 'a complete, operational system existing in living organisms which controls such basic functions as growth, healing and biological cycles'. He went on to describe the system in anatomical detail, describing its functions as 'a data transmission system in an analog fashion using varying levels of direct current as its signal. The system interlocks physically with the nervous system and is postulated to be its precursor. There are two electrochemical links of great significance in the operation of the system. One is between the DC system and the nervous system; the other is between the DC system and all body cells. The concept explains all of the diverse effects reported for the biological effects of applied electrical currents including: electrical anaesthesia, *electrical growth control and electroacupuncture.* It also furnishes a testable hypothesis for predicting other effects that might be of clinical significance'[11] (my italics).

In a personal communication with Dr Becker regarding my own research, he said:

'I am enclosing a copy of the paper presented in France and also a preprint of our specific data on acupuncture. Neither of these is up to date and we are vigorously pursuing this line of investigation at the present time. Our additional data, not reflected in either manuscript, has been supportive of our original conception and I believe at this time that I can unequivocally state that there are significant electrical correlations for approximately 50 per cent of the acupuncture points. We have concluded therefore, that acupuncture has a basis in reality. Our concept as briefly outlined in the French Symposium paper is that there is a previously undescribed system of data transmission additional to the nerves in living organisms. We believe that this system is primitive in nature, operates with analog type DC electrical signals and is concerned with the sensing of injury and effecting its control by healing processes. We believe the system is located in the perineural cells, Schwann cells peripherally and Glia cells centrally. There is evidence at least in the glia that these cells are capable of controlling the operational level of the nerve cells themselves. In this sense then, the system becomes analogous to a hybrid computor; that is, with a basic analog system and a superimposed high speed digital system. Since the primary input to the system is the sensing of injury, we postulate that this system, at least in part, carries the pain sensation. Since our data indicate that the

11 *Bioelectrochemistry and Bioenergetics,* Vol. 1, pp. 467–479.

system is electronic in nature, and carries messages by means of extremely small currents, the insertion of metallic needles could well produce significant perturbation. Of course, one can theoretically optimize the effect by the direct injection of electrical current.'

Chapter Five

Present State of Treatment

Following a number of papers on acupuncture anaesthesia in Western journals, a series of experiments was conducted with voltage-current measurements of acupuncture points 'lung 9' and adjacent 'liver 8'.[1]

Electrical significance of acupuncture points

The test employed was one that had already been described by Ann Woolley-Hart,[2] in which the current-voltage characteristics of the skin were measured. It had been observed that ohmic conditions prevailed until the point was reached where an increase in applied voltage led to a disproportionate increase in the observed current. This observation led to the concept that there is a threshold value of current, above which a change in tissue occurs.

In her conclusions Ann Woolley-Hart said:

'It would therefore seem that the acupuncture points "liver-8" and "lung 9" represent areas of skin that in diseased states of the relevant organs show altered functional properties. These changed properties are non-specific with regard to the skin and can be demonstrated by electrical tests which show, at specific sites, different current or resistence values compared with adjacent skin areas.'

However, this conclusion has been contested by other re-

1 J. Otto Bergman, MD, Austria, Ann Woolley-Hart, Department of Physics, The Polytechnic of Central London, 'Differences in Electrical Skin Conductivity Between Acupuncture Points and Adjacent Skin Areas', *The American Journal Of Acupuncture*, Vol. 1, January to March 1973.

2 'Some Physical and Physiological Aspects of the Passage of an Electric Current Through the Skin', *British Journal of Clinical Hypnosis*, Vol. 3, No. 4, October 1972.

searchers:[3]

'. . . It is concluded that no evidence whatsoever has been produced on the basis of which even the mere existence of electro-acupuncture points might be argued. All observations can be explained within the framework of biomechanical properties of the skin-electrode system . . .'

But this seemed an over-confident conclusion from an admittedly limited experiment, for still other researchers in other countries were conducting further experiments.[4]

Stimulation of animals

The use of electrodes for 'stimulation' (stimulating currents in animals had been applied for some years) has from the beginning had the implicit idea that these could reproduce physiological activity. A peripheral nerve thus stimulated would produce muscular contraction, or activate the sensory side of a reflex. Stimulation of the exposed surface of the motor cortex provided some of the earliest localizing information regarding function of that part of the brain's surface.

There was every reason, therefore, for the idea of stimulation to be firmly implanted in medical thinking, even though the results of these stimulating techniques were far from normal physiological actions.

A leader article in *The Lancet* (September 1974), discussing the 'sheer technical trickery' of the possibility of an implanted electrode being used to dictate normal functioning in an individual through remote control, concluded:

'There seems to be no reason why not. When Delgado, using such stimulation, stopped a charging bull in gallop, what was arresting was not only the bull's deceleration, but also the fact that the bull's rage was turned off (instead he indulged in mild displacement activities). It looked as though a true physiological

[3] Abraham Noordergraaf and Dennis Silace, 'Electro-Acupuncture', *IEEE Transaction on Biomedical Engineering*, September 1973.

[4] Dr Robert O. Becker, MD, Medical Investigator, Veterans Administration Hospital, New York, 'Electrical Correlations of Acupuncture Points', *Journal of Bioelectrochemistry and Bioenergetics*.

effect had been produced on the animal's behaviour. The limbic lobe, which has taken over automatic and emotional or temperamental functions, acts in a simple on-off way over a long time-scale, and seems eminently suitable for true stimulation. Although many parts of it have been stimulated acutely, our knowledge of the possibilities of long-term stimulation has hardly begun, despite the fact that Delgado and co-workers have made many investigations on animals, including primates, and even on a few human beings . . .'

Importance of form of electrical current

The same *Lancet* leader went on to describe a report of a case of spontaneous pain arising from a 'predominantly cortical' lesion and relieved by intermittent electrical stimulation through an electrode stereotaxically implanted in or near the internal capsule.

'The temporal cortex, as in all reported cases of this sort, was known to be damaged and the patient showed loss of right-parietal activity—that is, of functions on the left side of the body. The stimulating electrode was reckoned to be in the posterior limb of the internal capsule. Bipolar stimulation with waves of 0.25 milliseconds, 100 to 150 per second, 1.5 to 2.5 volts, produced a sensation of light tingling and vibration. After five to fifteen minutes, pain and an unpleasant spreading dysaesthesia disappeared, to remain at bay for one to twenty-six hours. *The exact form of the electrical current is important.* With these characteristics and the symptoms experienced by the patient it is likely that true stimulation was produced . . .' (my italics).

G. Douth, in his experimental cerebellar stimulation by implanted electrodes in cats[5] came to the conclusion, in studying the effects of different frequencies, train durations and pulse durations, that there exist optimal values for each of these parameters—although an increase in pulse duration may compensate for a deficiency in train duration; also that exceeding particular

[5] Proceedings of a symposium 'The Cerebellum, Epilepsy and Behaviour', held at St Barnabus Hospital, New York, August 1973.

values may provide no greater benefit to the patient. He further suggests that progressively larger currents recruit progressively larger populations of neurons, yet warns against using excessive current application.

Again, R. R. Myers and R. G. Bickford[5] demonstrated in both chloralose and sound induced myoclonus in cats, that cerebellar stimulation at frequencies of 100-200 cps clearly suppressed the myoclonus, whereas it was unaffected by stimulation at 1-10 cps. In Dr Cooper's patient with severe action myoclonus of 3 years' duration, a sequel of cerebral anoxia, there was no improvement for the first few weeks after implantation and stimulation at 200 cps. But improvement came gradually, and within a few months of continuous stimulation, her totally incapacitating generalized intention myoclonus had virtually disappeared.

Possible enduring neuro-chemical changes

I am reluctant at this early stage to provide a detailed account of my own investigations, which should more properly come at the end of my two-year period of research. But after approximately one year in London—the first six months of which were almost exclusively devoted to developing a machine that would provide a satisfactory current, wave-forms and frequencies—I have reached some broad conclusions over a fairly varied field.

My clinical findings to date parallel the conclusions of Dr Cooper (in a personal communication) in that electrical stimulation would appear to lead to enduring neuro-chemical changes. In the course of time it may well be proved, from clinical evidence emerging, that there is actual regeneration of neurones or, at least, a reconditioning of some brain circuits, such as the reticular formation. Significantly it has now been established[6] that in patients suffering from both endogenous and neurotic depression, the levels of cyclic AMP (adenosine cyclic monophosphate) are reduced. In these patients, urine level of cyclic AMP can be

6 *British Journal of Psychiatry*, Vol. 126, January 1975, p. 49.

restored to normal by electro-convulsive therapy. I hope to establish that the cyclic AMP can equally well be restored by longer term neuro-electric therapy, thus avoiding the undesirable side-effects of ECT and also the risks of addiction to mood-elevating drugs.

Electrical activity in damaged nerves

Writing in *Nature*[7] Drs Wall and Gutnick describe how damaged nerves attempt to regenerate. The nerve membrane changes its properties, becomes spontaneously active, and may be the source of pains. These impulse generators have unusual properties. They become silent after high frequency activity, and this silence, they say, may partially explain the effect of counter-stimulation as a pain therapy.

One of their conclusions regarding therapeutic implications related to electrical stimulation:

'Of more immediate interest is the use of electrical stimulation of peripheral nerves for the control of pain . . . It was shown that certain patients were relieved of their pain not only during the tetanic submaximal stimulation of their peripheral nerves but for long periods after the end of the stimulation whereas other patients were relieved only during stimulation . . .

'It may be that the prolonged relief which occurred in patients with damage to peripheral nerves was not produced by central inhibition but by the antidromic invasion of the damaged nerve which contained fragile generators of impulses of the type reported here . . . There is considerable physiological evidence that central inhibitions are generated by repetitive peripheral nerve stimulation . . .

Different reactions in electrical stimulation with different drugs

I am finding that there is a significant difference between treating local pain (sciatica, frozen shoulder, etc.) and the various addic-

7 Patrick D. Wall and Michael Gutnick, 'Properties of Different Nerve Impulses originating from a Neuroma', Vol. 248, 26 April 1974, pp. 740–743.

tions. In the cases of local pain, once the appropriate frequency is determined, there is probably little or no variation. In addiction the satisfactory frequencies change from individual to individual, often change in each individual from day to day, and even from treatment to treatment.

This would seem to indicate that Becker's theory of the data-bank biological control system—in addition to the nervous system—working like an analog computer is correct in suggesting that the body only absorbs the amount of electrical stimulation it requires for its immediate purpose and rejects the rest. This would also seem to be confirmed by the inhibiting effect of certain drugs on patients who are under neuro-electric treatment, with the potentiating effects of a few other drugs.

This signal-seeking device in turn would appear to be what Melzack describes as a 'central biasing mechanism' (located in a portion of the brainstem reticular formation).[8] It certainly makes sense of many of my earlier clinical observations which puzzled me, but which happened repeatedly as a result of neuro-electric therapy.

When heroin and methadone addicts commence therapy I prefer to stop all their drugs immediately, and give no substitution drugs whatever—not even linctus physeptone. One registered addict who was on a very high dosage of heroin and linctus physeptone took three days' dosage within three hours of beginning therapy. She did not even receive tranquillizers or sleeping pills, yet 48 hours later she went ice-skating at her own suggestion.

At present I withdraw barbiturate addicts gradually, as I have not yet established which frequency can be relied on to prevent withdrawal convulsions. But two heavily addicted cases who stopped all their barbiturates without informing me did not have any convulsions. Both patients had experienced withdrawal convulsions previously when being treated by other methods.

I still have not fully established which drugs potentiate and

[8] Ronald Melzack, *The Puzzle of Pain*, pp. 168, 199.

which depress effectiveness of neuro-electric stimulation (the Chinese claim that reserpine potentiates and atropine depresses the analgesic effect of finger acupuncture). However, I have observed that patients who take a single dose of various drugs during a course of neuro-electric therapy have diminished 'good' effects from that drug, and often quite an adverse reaction. One addict of 10 years' habituation drank a bottle of Codeine Syrup during therapy (quite a small dosage for him) and the effect, he volunteered, was like an I.V. dose of Apomorphine (which he had experienced previously as an aversive treatment). Another addict who injected large doses of cocaine intravenously while he was under treatment, found that neither the cocaine nor the machine had any effect.

This may provide a possible explanation for the more rapid cures observed in Hong Kong than I have experienced since my return to England in late 1973. In Hong Kong all our patients, including British and American, were admitted to the surgical and neuro-surgical wards of a free Hospital (no private hospital in Hong Kong, as in Britain, will accept a drug addict as a patient because of their disruptive and demanding characteristics), and no drugs were given to the patient, even in the first few difficult days of therapy when they were psychologically agitated and apprehensive. Most addicts in Britain will not tolerate this, and I believe that the administration of sedative and tranquillizing drugs slows down the neuro-chemical effects of the electric stimulation. Addicts treated recently have been more willing to refrain from tranquillizing drugs, and their response to therapy has been considerably more rapid. The only sedative drug I have found so far, which is definitely not counteracted by the electric stimulation, is oral Paraldehyde. On the other hand, I have not yet established whether or not Paraldehyde slows down the effect of the therapy. I suspect that it does.

Another interesting effect noticed in recent treatment of alcoholics is that if they have a relapse into drinking during therapy, they have a severe reaction from a much smaller amount of alcohol than in previous experience. Also, they do not seem to have the desire to drink again in order to remove the bad effects of their alcoholic bout (the 'hair of the dog' syndrome), as they would have done previously. This naturally suggests it may be possible to return to 'social drinking'. But at this stage in my research I give no indication of this possibility to the patient and urge them all to refrain from all alcoholic beverages, especially as many of them live so far away from treatment. Nevertheless, the Medical Council on Alcoholism recently published an article which suggested that many more alcoholics might be prepared for treatment if the aim was controlled drinking, instead of no drinking.[9] Neuro-electric therapy may well be a major step towards achieving controlled drinking. But intensive counselling would be required simultaneously with the therapy, to enable patients to find solutions to the problems which drove them into alcoholism in the first place.

Pocket-size stimulator for home use

I have developed a pocket-size stimulator so that suitable patients can continue treatment at home. The patient must be reasonably intelligent and motivated to continue his treatment at home, and must also report regularly for counselling and supervision.

One disadvantage of the pocket-size machine is that its range of wave-forms and frequencies is of necessity very limited compared to the larger machine. But the manufacturers state that they can pre-set these small machines to any medically recommended frequencies within a small range. This machine—the '530'—has only a rectangular wave-form and no modulation. Its pulse width range is .02 to 0.4 msec and frequency range 3 to 125 cps.

Frequency range in various conditions

Basically, depressive patients respond to a higher frequency (cps) and tense patients to lower frequencies, which definitely have a calming, relaxing effect so that patients frequently fall asleep during a treatment.

9 'Social Drinking as a Therapeutic Goal in the Treatment of Alcoholism', *The Journal of Alcoholism*, Vol. 9, No. 2, p. 43.

Also, addicts to narcotics and sedatives usually respond best within the frequency range of 75 to 300 cps; amphetamine addicts within 1000 to 2000 cps. Cigarette addicts respond to 5–10 cps but often need 2000 cps to break them from the final 3–4 cigarettes daily. Alcoholics generally respond to the lower ranges. One patient who was heavily addicted to hashish responded to 70 cps. If there are double addictions or concomitant physical illnesses, then the problem is more complex.

However I noticed recently that two of my heroin addict patients who are experts in electronic music were always changing the frequency at which I had set the machine. When I questioned them about this they said, 'This frequency just *feels* right.' I then tried the same method for my own migraines—going through the whole range of frequencies until I felt that one was 'right'—and found this to be a much more satisfactory method than just trying out different frequencies for different attacks.

I now allow most of my patients, once they have become accustomed to the treatments, to help decide the most effective frequency. Some are incapable of doing this but others, perhaps those more sensitive to sound, are very sure which is their 'correct' frequency. This 'correct' frequency usually varies, as I have said before, from treatment to treatment. For example, I usually give drug addicts a very low frequency for their last treatment when they retire to bed, to help them sleep.

Caution must be used with the higher frequencies, as they can cause both physical and mental agitation. Three people who were familiar with the effects of marijuana volunteered the observation that high frequencies made them feel as if they had smoked a joint of marijuana. None of these however, have continued to seek this treatment in order to produce these effects. In other words, no one has shown any sign of becoming addicted to or dependent on the machine so far.

Dr Irving Cooper reasoned from his scientific reading and research, that in cerebellar stimulation for epilepsy 10 cps should be used and for spastic conditions 200 cps. However, after finding that one epileptic who was unaffected by a cerebellar implant with a 10 cps frequency had his seizures totally controlled by 200 cps, Dr Cooper concluded that there is no set pattern of frequencies for different diseases.

Intensity of treatment

Since we cannot estimate the actual amount of electricity which reaches the brain, we have judged empirically that adequate voltage is being given when the patient has turned up the voltage sufficiently to allow him to feel a steady, pleasant tingling in his ears—sometimes it feels stronger in one ear than in the other, depending on the positioning of the electrodes. However, in my own migraines, I often feel that the pain is eased most when I turn up the voltage sufficiently to cause my occipital muscles to go into clonic spasm—not, by the way, a painful procedure. One hashish addict, in her second treatment, turned up the voltage until most of her scalp muscles were contracting strongly and said afterwards that she felt as if her 'brain had been cleansed'.

The average voltage used by patients is between 5 and 35 volts but this has to pass the resistance of skin, fascia, bone and dura. If a higher voltage is needed, it usually indicates that the batteries are becoming low, although a red light is provided on the machine to indicate when it is essential to renew the batteries. There is absolutely no danger of giving too high a voltage (the machine is run on batteries only), and even if the highest voltage were turned on (70 volts) it would only cause pain that was merely unpleasant.

Duration of treatment

When treating heroin and opium addicts in Hong Kong who were actually showing acute withdrawal symptoms, we noticed that the signs of withdrawals began to diminish about 15 minutes after the beginning of treatment. In another 5 or 10 minutes, the patients would occasionally fall asleep. So that in a total of some 30 minutes they were comfortable and happy. We therefore set 30 minutes as a recommended time for any one treatment. But I have since increased this to a basic 40 minutes for out-patient treatment.

I encourage in-patients who are alcoholics or drug addicts to keep the machine on as long as they can tolerate it, and, in particular, to keep it on when they go to sleep at night, as this seems to give them a more restful sleep. Their ears would be too uncomfortable if they kept the machine on for 24 hours a day, but, judging from the results of Dr Cooper's implanted pacemaker, the optimum would be continuous stimulation for the period of therapy. In no condition have I yet attempted to find the minimum necessary duration of therapy, but most of the drug addicts I have treated so far have succeeded in staying off their drugs after a shorter period of therapy than I had anticipated and have remained drug-free for up to one year, amongst those whom I have been able to follow-up in England.

Of three cases who left before completion of therapy and resorted to drug-taking, two returned later for further treatments. The reason for their lapses I attributed to lack of sufficient motivation, because they were basically more interested in being delivered from the serious consequences of their heavy addictions —e.g. physical, financial, domestic or social—than in being cured. I have tentatively concluded from experience with addicts who were not interested in coming off their addiction—but who submitted to family and other pressures—yet were eventually cured, that motivation of itself is not very important. But it must certainly be sufficient to accept the discipline of the full course of therapy.

I explain to the patients that therapy must continue until the craving for the drug or alcohol has completely disappeared. Because one can only accept the patient's word for it that there is no craving, I strongly recommend continuing therapy for a full 4 weeks. If this is not acceptable to the patient, I encourage him to return immediately for another few out-patient treatments if even a slight craving returns.

Patients are not likely to take treatment regularly if not under the doctor's supervision. But if they insist on leaving the hospital or clinic, then they should at least be encouraged to obtain a pocket-size stimulator and continue their own therapy at home. This is not ideal, but it is preferable to no treatment at all. One advantage of the 'home machine' is that if there should ever be a return of the craving the addict or alcoholic can treat himself immediately, without having to wait for an appointment with a doctor.

Treatment of pain

Several addicts who have come to me for treatment have become addicted to drugs because of chronic pain, which means treating their pain as well as their addiction.

Only two of these cases have had generalized pain and these showed a good response to treatment through the ears. One is a case of multiple sclerosis of 18 years' duration who uses the home-machine twice every day. After 3 months of therapy she reported that, although the machine would not stop an acute attack of pain (I am hoping that in further experimentation with frequencies, a method of at least diminishing acute pain will emerge), the incidence of pain was définitely much less than it had been for the previous 7 years, and that now she hardly ever took her pain-killers.

The second case was an otherwise healthy young woman of 33 who had had an acute onset of rheumatoid arthritis (confirmed serologically) 4–5 months previously. She was in this country for a few days only, but was desperate with pain, and refused to take any 'artificial medicines', including aspirin. With only 3 treatments, the pain was markedly reduced and the swelling of her wrist-joints obviously diminished, although it had not disappeared.

For all other cases I have used local application of electrical stimulation, as described by Nathan and Wall[10] and currently being used and investigated at the National Hospital for Nervous Diseases by Dr P. Nathan and Dr J. Bates. I and other are still

[10] Nathan and Wall, 'Treatment of Post-Herpetic Neuralgia by Prolonged Electric Stimulation', *British Medical Journal*, 1974, Vol. 3, pp. 645–647.

experimenting with different types of flat electrodes for distal use.

The Chinese method of determining the area of stimulation by measuring alterations in the electrical resistance of the skin, may well be of significance in the optimum area of applying electrodes, as well as for inserting acupuncture needles. The altered spontaneous currents associated with the onset of an attack of pain also deserve investigation.

Cases of frozen shoulder can, with a few treatments, be given complete freedom from pain and markedly improved movement. Pain due to trauma, or division of nerves, or pressure on nerves, requires a great deal of thought and investigation to find the correct area for application of the electrodes. Such cases also need repeated, sometimes almost continuous, treatments, and only time will tell if the electrical stimulation will eventually be actually curative.

The only type of headache I have treated so far is the migraine headache, and in this the frequency of the current is very important. I have not yet collected enough figures to make data significant, but my impression is definitely that the optimum frequency must be found by the patient and that the treatment should continue for about 1½ hours. Chinese acupuncturists claim to arrest migraines with a few seconds of needling, but by using electro-stimulation the headache and other symptoms gradually diminish over a period of a few hours. However, the neuro-electric treatment, although slower than acupuncture, does not need to be repeated even though the attack is due to last a few days. Moreover, treatment by acupuncture tends to become less effective with time,[11] whereas with neuro-electric stimulation the incidence of migraines steadily diminishes.

Summary of investigations

There is no doubt that one treatment with electro-acupuncture, for 20 to 40 minutes, *without the administration of any drugs at all,*

11 Personal Communication from the Migraine Trust.

will dramatically alleviate the symptoms of acute withdrawal in any drug addiction, in the same way as it relieves the bronchial spasm of status asthmaticus.[12] This would indicate that the neuro-electric stimulation affects the autonomic nervous system directly and rapidly. I personally have witnessed the effects in both conditions many times, even when an addict, for example, is in the severest withdrawals. Many other drugs can relieve withdrawal symptoms, but I know of no other treatment that will bring such immediate relief without the use of drugs.

Another outstanding feature of this type of therapy is that, in addition to having his physical symptoms eased, the addict becomes immediately responsive to behavioural therapy. Dr Maurice Sainsbury of the New South Wales Institute of Psychiatry, Australia, points out, of one patient whom he treated by Dr Wen's original method, 'She has been able to take part in the ward programme without being "bombed out" for some days.'[13]

But it should be stressed that intensive challenging and supportive therapy must be given immediately the treatment is begun, because by this method the patient seems to be more immediately aware of himself—his faults, his personal problems, the future problems of living without drugs and, most important of all, his alienation—than with other methods of withdrawal. But the relief he obtains from the neuro-electric therapy provides an unpressured opportunity in which to consider alternative solutions to those problems.

Even this has its dangers, as there are often temporary phases of euphoria (the first phase usually occurs a few days after the commencement of therapy and the second after 10 days) which have to handled very carefully, because the patient tends to become over-confident and feels that no more therapy is required. The full month's therapy is necessary, even though some patients respond more rapidly than others, and a further six weeks'

[12] See p. 33.

[13] Maurice J. Sainsbury, Letter to *The Medical Journal of Australia*, June 1, 1974; 'Acupuncture in Heroin Withdrawal,' *The Medical Journal of Australia*, 1974, 2: 102–105.

rehabilitative convalescence is recommended, when the patient should be encouraged to take up some form of outside physical work as employment therapy, as well as other activities.

However, the more vital question of whether this therapy removes the *craving* for the drug permanently can only be measured statistically over many years of careful follow-up. At present, only the addict's assurance of craving removal, together with his obviously changed demeanour, can be used as evidence—apart from that provided by family and friends regarding the improvement in the patient's condition and character. This latter improvement is often quite dramatic.

In Hong Kong both Chinese and European patients declared that any one treatment would take away their craving for 1 to 2 hours in the first 2 to 4 days of therapy. This sudden 'freedom from craving' with the first treatment has been claimed by only a few drug addicts treated since my return to England, but it has been experienced by several alcoholics and cigarette smokers—the effects of a single treatment lasting from 24 to 48 hours in the case of alcohol and nicotine.

In Britain, while many addicts come seeking this therapy, many of them have deep-seated resistance to being cured, either because it is part of their desired life-style or because they are unwilling to face up to the demands of the 'real' world. It may also be because they are reluctant to lose the drug they describe as 'a friend'. Despite this resistance, I have proved that they can still be successfully treated. But because of it I sometimes give them additional sedative and tranquillizing drugs (not the drug of their addiction) to persuade them to complete the therapy, although I prefer to stop all drugs as soon as possible. In such cases the 'freedom from craving' comes quite suddenly at some point after two to four weeks (as opposed to ten days to two weeks in those who do not receive any drugs at all). They describe this feeling as 'being let out of prison'.

To date, I am finding that alcoholics respond better to outpatient treatment while living in their own homes and being helped to deal with their domestic situations at the same time as undergoing their therapy. Unlike the typical drug addict, the alcoholic usually has specific problems from which he chooses to escape through alcohol, and he must learn that he can cope with those problems without having to resort to the escape of alcoholic oblivion. The therapy appears to help alcoholics considerably in providing the optimism that they can cope.

On the other hand, there is no doubt that the therapy works better when the drug of addiction is cut off completely, but usually this cannot be done with out-patients. Only a very few are sufficiently motivated to stop the drug totally when controlling it themselves. But in Britain there are approximately 300,000 alcoholics and even more addicts to barbiturates, tranquillizers and pain-killers, and most of them can be helped only as out-patients.

The Chinese report that anaesthetised animals under general anaesthesia do not respond to acupuncture, and my clinical impression would seem to confirm this, in that neuro-electric therapy is less effective and slower in action when the patient continues to take drugs. To establish this pattern more clearly, I am conducting a pilot project at one of the National Health Service Drug Dependence Units, treating a few addicts, selected at random, with one treatment three times weekly for a period of six months. Each addict treated will be assessed by a psychiatrist at the beginning and end of the course of therapy.

The addicts are being asked to reduce their dosage of drugs when they feel they can cope with a smaller amount. The dishonesties of addiction (e.g. selling 'spare' drugs to get money for food, cinema, cigarettes, etc.) will make it difficult to get accurate results, but it should at least indicate the value or otherwise of the out-patient method. If its efficacy should be established, it will not be very time-consuming, since anyone of average intelligence learns how to put on the electrodes and adjust the controls (under medical guidance) after two or three treatments. The Shackman-Patterson stimulator can be supplied with several outlets to treat four patients simultaneously with individual output control. But it is probably better to use individual stimulators to allow for different frequencies in different patients.

The outcome of this out-patient pilot project will be reported as soon as it is completed.

No addict to compulsive gambling has been treated, but it is hoped to do a pilot study in this field, because in theory the compulsion and addiction is similar. A medical colleague using this therapy for compulsive eating claims to be getting an encouraging response in two cases, but I have not personally treated this form of addiction.

Side effects

On a few occasions a patient has complained of headaches, and even nausea, when the 'wrong' frequency has been used, but a change of frequency can eliminate these side effects. Apart from this, side effects have been few and either of no significance (e.g., improvement of hair texture) or actually beneficial. Some patients have experienced an increase in sexual desire and potency, even in cases other than addiction. An improvement in sleep is often reported.

When the craving disappears, character improvements are frequently marked, either as a direct result of the therapy, or as a side effect from the freedom from the drugs, or alcohol, or both. Tensions are lessened and there is a definite alleviation of depression, which would suggest that treatment of post-addiction psychoses should be possible.

Chapter Six

Rehabilitation Treatments: Some Spiritual Aspects

No discussion of the treatment of drug addiction would be complete without some mention of the important part played by spiritual values in restructuring the life of the addict in rehabilitation treatment. But since this is even more important than the purely medical treatment—in that it provides the foundation on which a new life can be built which will obviate the need to resort to drugs—a follow-up book is needed, and already in hand, to deal with the subject more fully. At first I thought that this spiritual rehabilitation aspect could be taken at the later, convalescent, stage. But it became obvious in the many varied patients I was treating that the related problems had to be treated concurrently, because of the rapidity with which the neuro-electric treatment brings them out of their drug-hazed state.

Relationship between drugs and the occult

The relationship between drugs and the mystical is established in the words the Greeks used, *pharmakos*, meaning drug, medicine, poison—and sorcery. For example, in the New Testament, *pharmakos* is used 'as an adjective signifying "devoted to magical arts"; is used as a noun, *sorcerer*, especially one who uses drugs, potions, spells, enchantments.'[1] In sorcery, the explanation continues, the use of drugs, whether simple or potent, was generally accompanied by incantations and appeals to occult powers, with provision of various charms, amulets, etc., professedly designed to keep the applicant or patient from the attention and power of demons, but actually to impress the appli-

1 W. E. Vine, *Expository Dictionary of New Testament Words*, Oliphants, London, pp. 51-2

cant with the mysterious resources and powers of the sorcerer.

At some point the drug addict—either because of drug usage, or because of an insatiable hunger for a more intense 'high', or because of an unconscious realization that no chemical can ever really replace the spiritual, which is his or her real hunger—begins to dabble in the occult ('that which involves the supernatural, mystical or magical') as a possible solution to the basic problem of alienation.

The sorcerer or witch-doctor has been consigned to history, along with demons and angels and 'the provision of various charms, amulets, etc.', but modern doctors prescribing drugs, *without* what may be called 'the X-factor of powers other than human' are now faced with a major problem: how long can they go on ignoring the mounting number of mental disorders, the proliferation of drug addicts and alcoholics, and ease their increasingly troubled consciences by prescribing the deadly barbiturates or other sedatives and tranquillizers which eventually only intensify the problem?

Doctors and the middle-aged to blame

Despite popular belief that it is only the young who are responsible for the soaring statistics of drug addiction, it is, in fact, mostly the middle-aged who are to blame—and the over-prescribing doctors, of course.

In 1970 there were 47.2 million prescriptions for psychotropic drugs—sleeping pills, appetite suppressants, tranquillizers and anti-depressants—issued in England and Wales alone. From 1965 to 1970 prescriptions for these drugs increased by 19 per cent, from 39.7 million to 47.2 million. During these six years 120 million prescriptions for hypnotic drugs were dispensed in England and Wales, and there was a remarkable shift from the barbiturate to the non-barbiturate hypnotics. These increased by 145 per cent, 'a figure entirely accounted for by the prescribing of two drugs (Mandrax and Mogadon) both introduced in 1965'.[2] Peter Parish described this widespread use of these agents

2 Peter Parish, *Drugs and Society*, April 1972.

as a 'pharmacological leucotomy on a large section of contemporary society'. The majority of those to whom these drugs go are not young people, Parish noted.

'Twice as many women as men received them and the number of patients of both sexes receiving these drugs increased rapidly from the age of eighteen to twenty-five. For women the increase continued up to the age of fifty and then levelled off until sixty-five when it rose again. By contrast there was a continued and progressive increase in the number of men receiving treatment from twenty-five to seventy-five years of age . . .'

It is of little comfort to know that historically the attractions of drugs are not new. Dr Richard H. Blum of Stanford University, California, a pioneer in the study of drugs and the author of several books on the subject, has written:

'One finds over the centuries men seeking—and drugs offering—health, relief of pain, security, mystical revelations, eternal life, the approval of the gods, relaxation, joy, sexuality, restraint, blunting of the senses, escape, ecstasy, stimulation, freedom from fatigue, sleep, fertility, the approval of others, clarity of thought, emotional intensity, self-understanding, self-improvement, power, wealth, degradation, a life philosophy, exploitation of others, enjoyment of others, value enhancement, and one's own or another's death'.[3]

Over the past few decades five themes of rehabilitation of the drug addict have emerged:

1. *communal*: resembling the homogeneity of the folk culture, with strong roots in face-to-face interaction;
2. *community interaction*: involving the addict with his given community;
3. *religion*: providing an intense religious experience for those willing to be saved, who are then expected to return to the community and become involved in saving other addicts;
4. *rational authority*: placing the addict on probation, if convicted of a crime, rather than sending him to prison;

[3] *Drugs and Society*, Jossey-Bass Publications Inc., San Francisco, 1969.

5. *chemotherapy*: such as methadone maintenance.

These are all still being used, either on their own or in combination. Before looking at the drug problem and its close religious associations, I will digress to comment on the difference between drug dependence and drug addiction.

Drug dependence and drug addiction

Drug-dependence is usually described as a state, caused by the taking of a drug, so that the stopping of the drug produces a disturbance; which, in turn, can only be stopped again by taking the initial drug, or one with which it is cross-dependent. Drug-dependence, therefore, describes the relationship between an individual and a drug.

But in contrast—and this is not always recognized—drug addiction is something different, and describes a relationship between a dependent individual and society, in that it leads to behaviour contravening social norms; for example, absence from or incompetence at work, stealing, or possessing drugs illicitly.

The most characteristic feature of disturbance produced by the dependent individual stopping the drug is a subjective condition known as 'drug hunger'. This usually takes the form of compulsive 'drug seeking', and may be measured in terms of the effort made, or the money spent, to obtain the lacking drug. This drug-hunger, and the efforts made to alleviate it, are evidence of *psychic dependence*.

The evidence of *physical* dependence is demonstrated by 'withdrawals' or body changes, such as sweating, tremors, diarrhoea and cramps, and so on—commonly known as 'the monkeys'.

It is important to separate the two sets of symptoms because *psychic* dependence is more important than the *physical*, for two reasons. First, every addictive drug induces psychic dependence, but only some induce physical dependence; second, some drugs such as nalorphine or corticosteroids that do not induce psychic dependence—even though they induce physical dependence—are not addictive.

Drugs and their mystical effects

The opiates (opium, morphine, heroin). Opium is a drug that has a venerable place in history and which has been in medical use as a pain-killer for at least 2,000 years, possibly for much longer. In addition to countering traumatic pain it was used in over-activity of the gut (dysentery, diarrhoeas) and inflammation of the respiratory tract. The application of opium simply to achieve pleasurable effects does not seem to have taken root before the end of the eighteenth century in China. Early in the nineteenth century a German chemist, Serturner, isolated the chief alkaloid of opium and produced morphine, from which was derived its more dangerous companion, heroin. Over two dozen other alkaloids have since been derived from opium, the best-known being codeine, used in cough remedies.

After experiencing the effects of opium De Quincey wrote:

'O heavens! What a revulsion! What a resurrection from its lowest depths, of the inner spirit! What an apocalypse of the world within me! That my pains had vanished was now a trifle in my eyes; this negative effect was swallowed up in the immensity of the positive effects which had opened up before me, in the abyss of divine enjoyment thus revealed. Here was a panacea for all human woes; here was the secret of happiness, about which the philosophers had disputed for so many ages, at once discovered . . .'

Marijuana group (grass, pot, cannabis, hash, etc.). New evidence about the effects of marijuana is now being produced every few months that would seem, on balance, to make it a more serious indulgence than was previously thought. While effects vary, the user who imbibes the smoke with as great a quantity of oxygen as possible usually experiences a transient euphoria with feelings of superiority and superhuman powers of insight. Sights and sounds become very vivid and very meaningful. There is a distortion of the user's sense of time and space, coupled with loss of judgement. At this point the will to act is severely restrained and the user experiences 'oneirocritic ecstasy', or 'blessed repose', during which the will to act is destroyed.

Marijuana produces a marked psychic dependence (*not* addictive) and has been summarized thus: 'Cannabis is a surprising drug that can make the impossible seem real and the real seem unnecessary.' In a report to the National District Attorney's Council on Drug Abuse (13 April, 1970) Dr Edward Bloomquist, MD, Associate Clinical Professor of Surgery (Anaesthesia), University of Southern California School of Medicine stated:

'The user gets hung up on a life cycle. This guy is as much a slave as the heroin junkie except for the physical results . . . There is an increased factor that influences a search for mystical religions along with a pre-occupation with the new morality. One can philosophize readily but logic is impaired. It alters the user's relation to reality. It removes kids from a rational religion.'

In India the use of hemp as 'bhang' or 'ganja' is widespread. What it offers as a flight from reality in that country has been well described by an ancient Indian writer:

'To the Hindu the hemp plant is holy. A guardian lives in the bhang leaf . . . Bhang is the Joy-Giver, the Sky-Flier, the Heavenly Guide, the Poor Man's Heaven, the Soother of Grief . . . No God or man is as good as the religious drinker of bhang. The students of the scriptures at Benares are given it before they sit to study. At Benares, Ujjain and other holy places, yogis, bairagis and sanyasis take deep draughts of bhang that they may centre their thoughts on the Eternal . . .'[4]

Cocaine (coke, snow, happy dust). 'Mama Coca' is one of the most famous names in Inca history, her name perpetuating the Quechua word for 'mother' and 'coca'—the divine plant of the Incas. The dangerous alkaloid from this magical leaf was isolated by a German chemist, Gaedeke, in 1885. In other words, cocaine bears the same relation to coca that nicotine does to tobacco—providing a threat that many choose to ignore. The wine of

4 Quoted in Norman Taylor, *Narcotics: Nature's Dangerous Gifts*, Dell Publishing Co. New York, 1970, p. 30.

coca made by Angelo Mariani was drunk by Pope Leo XIII, and made Mariani a huge fortune, and the soft drink Coca Cola included it as one of the original ingredients (now forbidden), making the company an even greater fortune.

The Incas used the coca leaf to give freedom from fatigue, but also being essentially religious they used it to provide exultation of spirit—and put it into burial urns to sustain the departed on their last journey.

Cocaine is an excitant, a stimulant almost immediately acting on the higher levels of the brain, so that the user is filled with a sense of increased mental and physical power. But the ecstatic uplifting of the ego does not last long and, when it goes, serious hallucinations and delusions of persecution take over. Cocaine can be stopped with only mild discomfort and depression, but when this is done too often—as, for instance, in the case of those who use it to overcome strains or accomplish demanding tasks—the effects can become disastrous. Convulsions often occur and mental deterioration takes place. The most extreme cases end as wretched and pathetic occupants of mental institutions.

Cocaine is responsible for the 'double addiction' problem, in that when the user stops the drug he often resorts to heroin to enable him to overcome the black depressions and nameless fears. From this combination the underworld derives the terms 'dynamite', 'speedball' and 'H and C'.

LSD (Acid). Under LSD the user can experience a variety of hallucinations, delusions, time and space distortions, abnormal body sensations and other deviations from normal consciousness. Dr A. E. Wilder Smith, DSc, PhD, DesSc, FRIC, Professor at the University of Illinois Medical Centre, Chicago, has declared:[5]

'Changes in thought follow a free flow of bizarre ideas . . . Some LSD adherents claim inspiration under the influence of the drug . . . the subconscious rises to the conscious level . . . Most of us live 70 years. The acid user lives a million years in a second. It is a highly intense thing—he not only talks with God, he *was*

[5] *The Drug Users*, Harold Shaw, Wheaton, Illinois, p. 63.

God. This religious thing has become a real thing . . .'

Wilder Smith goes on to record the experience of a chronic alcoholic who was hospitalized, given LSD, and who previously had had very little experience of religion:[6]

'I found myself drifting into another world . . . I saw a gleaming, blinding light with a brilliance no man has ever known. It had no shape or form, but I *knew* I was looking at God Himself . . . All of a sudden I was back in eternity . . . Peace and happiness and tranquillity . . . My heart was filled with a joy that was overwhelming . . .

'There must have been a short pause in the music, but to me it seemed an eternity. I said, "Don't stop it. God is whole in me." At this point I felt as if God were holding me in His arms and revealing himself to me. I smiled and said, "I've found him, I've found him!" I had such a tremendous sense of peace and well-being. After so many years of running alone and afraid, God was now with me.'

Another, non-Christian, writer, Dr Timothy Leary, a convert to Hinduism, who has been called 'the father of drugs', has said that psychedelic experience is fundamentally a religious experience—transcendentally oriented.

'The instruments of systematic religion are chemicals . . . All Drugs are the religion of the 21st century. Pursuing the religious life today without using psychedelic drugs is like studying astronomy with the naked eye . . . Man is so sick . . . that today it is safe to say that drugs are the specific and almost the only way that America is going to have a religious experience.'[7]

Religion is ecstasy, states Leary, and this is the main emphasis of the psychedelic drug revolution—not escapism and not drugs *per se*.

Alcohol. In the past it has been said that the behaviour of alcoholics indicates a search for the spiritual—they search for God inside a bottle. But Dr Pierre Fouquet, Consultant to the World Health Organisation, repudiates this assertion and states:

6 Ibid., p. 42.

7 *Politics of Ecstasy*, Putnam, New York, 1968, pp. 157–293.

'On the contrary, a return to a religion, of whatever sort, could constitute a powerful weapon in individual therapy or mass prophylaxis.'[8]

But in a remarkable work, published in 1936, a Protestant pastor, Dr Felice, under the provoking title, *Holy Poisons, Divine Drunkenness*, treats alcoholism and drug addiction together, and writes of pathological drinkers:

'They are votaries of a particular kind who perform unconsciously certain rituals which will open to them another world—a supernatural world. After all, why do so many human beings deliberately expose themselves to the dangers of poisons? It is that here again come into play needs, desires and traditions which show their religious character . . .'[9]

To support his thesis he cites the opinions of such authors as William James (*The Religious Experience*), Leuba (the mystical experience obtained by material means in *Psychology of Religious Mysticism*), and Bergson (*The Two Sources of Morals and Religion*).

There is little doubt that alcohol has played an important role in the spiritual history of mankind and in the main religions. And in the twentieth century alcohol is the main psychotropic drug in the world, whether used in primitive or civilised communities. The religious use of alcohol has always been endowed with high spiritual meaning, even when this meaning was distorted or abused. The apostle Paul in the New Testament (Ephesians 5:18) notes the significant similarity and significant difference in the alcoholic and religious experiences when he writes: 'Be not drunk with wine, wherein is excess; but be filled with the Spirit.'

Some significant treatments of addiction

Transcendental Meditation (TM). Transcendental Meditation has been claimed to be one answer to the problem of drug addiction and abuse. The cult—if that is the word—of TM was brought to

[8] *Notes on Alcohol and Alcoholism*, Medical Council on Alcoholism, Chapter XXIII, 1974.

[9] 'Philosophical Religious Factors in Alcoholism', *Quarterly Journal of Studies in Alcoholism*, 24, 1963, pp. 473-488.

the West by the Maharishi Mahesh Yogi, was briefly espoused by the Beatles, and has since become something of a vogue in the United States and Britain—and a subject for scientific investigation.

It is not a religion, but a technique for relaxation which can be learned easily and which centres on a 20-minute period of meditation in the morning and a similar period in the evening.

One of the most interesting pieces of research which has so far been carried out into the effects of this technique concerns 2,000 student meditators, of whom 68 per cent were admitted drug users.[10] After six months TM only 35 per cent were still using marijuana, and after 21 months this figure had dropped to only 12 per cent. Nearly half of the students (940) admitted that they used LSD before starting TM. At the end of the 21-month survey period only 3 per cent were doing so. Over the same period dependence on alcohol and tobacco was reduced to two-thirds.

Students who had given up the use of drugs claimed that TM improved their sense of well-being and mental alertness to such a degree that they felt no need of artificial stimuli.

Transactional Analysis (TA). In his book, *I'm OK—You're OK: A Practical Guide to Transactional Analysis*,[11] T. A. Harris describes Transactional Analysis as both a teaching and learning device. He describes four life positions underlying people's behaviour:

1. *I'm not OK—You're OK*, which is the anxious dependence of the immature.
2. *I'm not OK—You're not OK*, showing the 'giver-up' or despair position.
3. *I'm OK—You're not OK*, indicating the criminal position.
4. *I'm OK—You're OK*, which is the response of the mature adult, at peace with himself and others.

Harris concludes that most people still operate unconsciously from the position, *I'm not OK—You're OK.*

10 *World Medicine*, Vol. 8, No. 25.

11 Harper and Row, New York, 1969.

The transaction consists of a stimulus by one person and a response by another, which in turn becomes a new stimulus for the other person to respond to. The purpose of the analysis is to discover which part of each person—parent, adult or child—is originating each stimulus and response.

Addicts on the TA programme receive group treatment and interaction, video-tape replay of the TA sessions, some vocational training, and are aided by 'linkers' who are themselves former addicts going between the authoritarian structure (warden, programme directors, employers) and other resident addicts.

Teen Challenge (TC). Teen Challenge (in the United States) is the most publicized of the 'Christian' programmes of treatment and is an organization founded by David Wilkerson, author of *The Cross and the Switchblade*,[12] to treat drug addicts. It scarcely qualifies, by accepted standards, as a therapeutic community and, in fact, it is opposed to conventional therapy sessions, not accepting that their group 'rap sessions'—prayer and Bible studies—are in any sense similar.

In a recent statistical study on the treatment of heroin addiction in the United States by Teen Challenge and the regime of Transactional Analysis, seventeen subjects were assigned at random to each of three treatment regimes: No Treatment (NT), Teen Challenge (TC) or Transactional Analysis (TA), with the subjects in the last two groups being under treatment for 6 to 12 months. The purpose of the experiment was to determine whether these approaches had a differential effect on heroin addiction. A score on a standardized questionnaire and recidivism (relapse) rates, measured over a 29-month period, were used as an index of the effectiveness of each treatment. The data, as measured by the criterion given, the questionnaire results and recidivism rates, gave unequivocal support for three findings:

1. that TC is an effective programme of treatment;
2. that TA is a very effective method of treatment;
3. that, based on the lower questionnaire score when compared

12 Published in Britain by Marshall, Morgan and Scott.

to NT and the lower recidivism rates, TA is the best regime of treatment for heroin addiction of. the three treatments investigated.

However, TA's rate of recidivism was found to be 100 per cent lower over a 2-9 month period than that of TC. Recidivism rates, computed from the TC and TA records and being defined as again returning to drugs, were for TC and TA programmes 32 per cent and 16 per cent respectively.[13]

The author's conclusion is well worth noting by all Christians working in the drug field:

'While it is true that the TC programme seems to help the addict increase his self-awareness, it is also true that the approach deals with heroin and other addictions in a repressive manner, i.e., the motivation of the addict had been changed because of his conversion to Christ whom he accepts as his Lord and Master and accordingly views drug-taking as a sin. It appears that dealing with heroin addiction in this manner masks the symptoms and aetiology, and in doing so does not get at the real causes which led up to the addict becoming addicted to heroin and other drugs. Thus, the addict's belief in Christ, even though sincere and real, becomes a drug substitution which often never grows beyond that little spark of embryonic faith . . .

'Addicts often have had a rather poor relationship with their earthly fathers. These negative feelings which come about as the result of the poor interpersonal relationship between father and addict could very well be carried over into the matter of their faith in Christ. Thus loss of faith would occur because the addict had only had a change of environment, conversion, undergone detoxification, and was now beginning to feel better because of regular hours, and eating habits. But the root causes which had allowed that individual addict to become addicted in the first place had not been acted upon in psychotherapy . . .'

Significantly, it was also concluded from the TC group scores that it seemed likely that the approach changes the addiction

13 G. Archie Johnston, 'Heroin Addiction. Teen Challenge vs. Transactional Analysis: A Statistical Study', *U.S. Journal of American Scientific Affiliation*, Vol. 25, No. 3, 1973.

concept in the addict's self-image rapidly at the point of his conversion, this change being based upon his faith in Christ.
It is this continuous and literal working-faith and the 'love of Christ' which controls him. However it was also concluded that if the addict did not fervently keep active in the TC programme, or in the church, he could encounter a personal loss of faith—even momentarily—which could result in his returning to drug-usage.

It is unfortunate that success of Christian values has been so closely identified with Teen Challenge and similar ultra-fundamentalist emphases. For there are other recent researches in England (not yet published) which demonstrate that there are basically different Christian approaches that produce significantly better results than any others reportedly yet achieved.

The necessity for spiritual values

Victor Frankl, founder of what has come to be known as the Third Viennese School of Psychiatry, has postulated that besides Freud's 'pleasure principle', and Adler's 'will to power', there exists yet another,—a 'will to meaning'—as an equally fundamental drive. He says:[14]

'It is an inherent tendency in man to reach out for meanings and for values to actualise. In contrast to animals, man is not told by his instincts what he must do. And in contrast to man in former times, he is no longer told by his traditions and values what he ought to do . . . Thousands and thousands of young students are exposed to an indoctrination along the lines of a reductionist concept of life which denies the existence of values . . . The result is a world-wide phenomenon—more and more patients are crowding our clinics with the complaint of an inner emptiness, the sense of a total and utter meaninglessness of life . . .'

This type of neurosis he calls 'noogenic', as distinct from sexual and other types of neuroses, and he claims that about 20 per cent of all cases at the Vienna Psychiatric Clinic (of which

[14] *Beyond Reductionism—The Alpach Syndrom*, edited by A. Koestler and J. R. Smythies, London, 1969.

he is the Director) are of noogenic origin. He further claims that this figure is doubled among student patients of Central European origin—and that it soars to 80 per cent among students in the United States.

Arthur Koestler, writing of this startling factor in *Protest and Discontent*[15] compares this mood of 'existential vacuum' caused by the frustration of 'the will to meaning' with 'the mood of the Pink Decade, the 1930's', when the western world was convulsed by economic depression, unemployment and hunger marches, and when the so-called 'Great Socialist Experiment' initiated by the Russian Revolution seemed to be the only hopeful ideal to a great mass of hopeful idealists, including himself. He writes:

'In *The God that Failed* I wrote about that period: "Devotion to pure Utopia and rebellion against polluted society are the two poles which provide the tension of all militant creeds. To ask which of the two makes the current flow—attraction by the ideal or repulsion by the social environment—is to ask the old question whether the hen was first or the egg."

'Compare this with the present mood. Today the repellant forces are more powerful than ever, but the attraction of the ideal is missing, since what we thought to be Utopia turned out to be a cynical fraud. The egg is there, but no hen to hatch it. Rebellion is free-wheeling in a vacuum . . .

'It is, of course, true that similar negative moods can be found in past periods of our history, variously described as *mal de siècle*, romantic despair, Russian nihilism, apocalyptic expectations. And there have been Ranters, Messianic sects and Tarantula dancers, all of whom have their striking contemporary parallels. But the present has a unique and unprecedented urgency because the rate of change is now moving along an ever steeper exponential curve, and history is accelerating like the molecules in a liquid coming to the boil . . .'

It would seem obvious, therefore, that any possible form of therapy for drug addictions (from the opioids through alcohol

15 Edited by Bernard Crick and William A. Robson, Penguin Books.

and nicotine to the barbiturates and amphetamines), caused to a great extent by the lack of this 'will to meaning' in the lives of the sufferers, must also take into consideration at an early stage the communication of a new set of spiritual values of a depth and scope not heretofore considered by doctors, if the patient is to be really cured of the condition that led him or her into addiction in the first place. In the present busy life of hospital, clinic or consulting-room this may not be possible, but consideration could be given to the setting up of clinics where medical, nursing and social worker staff could be integrated into a single unit treating all of the drug addicts', including alcoholics', problems spiritually as well as medically. It is no longer necessary to prove that a society which neglects the former in favour of the latter does so at its peril.

What became quickly apparent—both in Hong Kong and London, with the remarkably quick effect of the treatment described earlier—was that the patients, so suddenly relieved of cravings as well as withdrawal symptoms, were left in a spiritual vacuum, a condition of inability to deal with the problems which had induced their addiction. They were thus only 'half-cured'. It was evident, therefore, that an environment was necessary in which they could be treated *medically* by the electrical stimulation; *spiritually* by nurses—male and female—who would be equipped to deal with the particular problems of the addict, or the neurologically disturbed; and *sociologically* by social workers in both short and long-term follow up—both medical and social workers themselves having an experience or knowledge of the spiritual values to communicate to their patients.

With all kinds of addicts now numbering millions; with doctors too hard-pressed to do more than increase doom-filled statistics of prescription-writing; and with some insurance and private hospital plans excluding drug addicts, alcoholics and the mentally disturbed from their benefits, this would seem a worthy medical enterprise in our own country, and an inspiring challenge to administrators, financiers, doctors, nurses and the socially concerned.

It would be only appropriate if, in crossing new frontiers of the mind medically, Christians in particular could bring back to healing the spiritual dimension that has been lost in recent history, through pioneering some form of clinic-community for treatment of the whole person.

Appendix I
Multi-purpose electro-therapeutic apparatus for Chinese acupuncture points (Model 'Shoi Wei' 6.26)

The instrument is battery powered (6 x HP11) and is contained in a transistor receiver case with carrying handle. It provides for the location of acupuncture points by audible indication of skin resistance and a choice of one of three stimulation outputs to the needles when inserted. Three patients can be treated simultaneously with separate intensity controls (transformer isolation).

The circuit comprises:

a) A basic blocking oscillator pulse generator and modulator/output stage.

b) A surging wave-form generator and buffer output to (a) when required.

c) Three individual output transformers and intensity controls.

d) Switched option of loudspeaker or neon lamp to indicate pulses or surges.

The maker's specification (electrical) is not published, or at least not available.

Functional Data
(from tests on single sample)

FUNCTION MODE SWITCH
Pos. 1 (anti-clockwise)
Surge modulated pulses adjustable from 0.4 to 10Hz (fails above 10Hz).

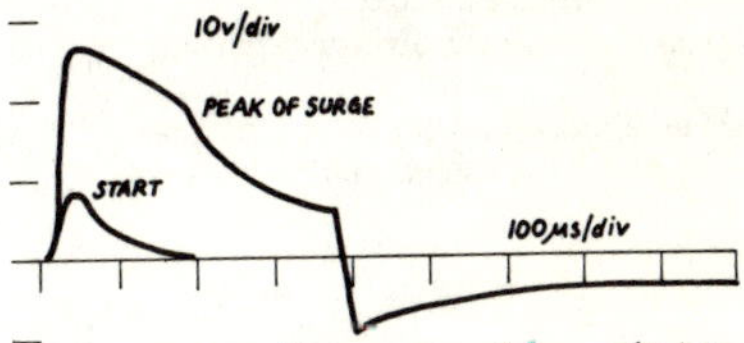

Pulse duration ms	*Frequency in Hz*	*Max. volts into specified load*
0.35 ms	70Hz	26 into 1K 36 into 2K 44 into 3K

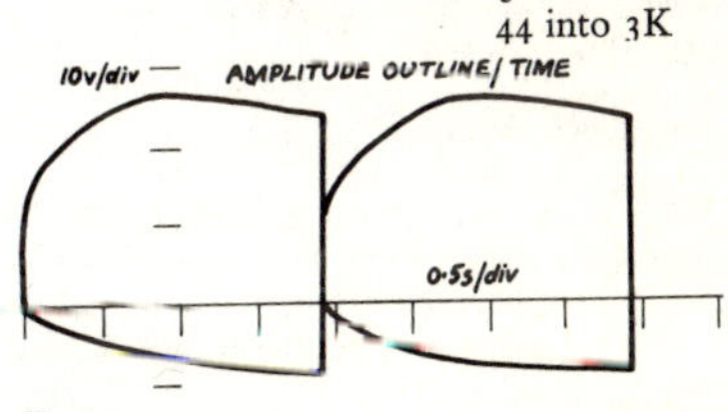

Pos. 2

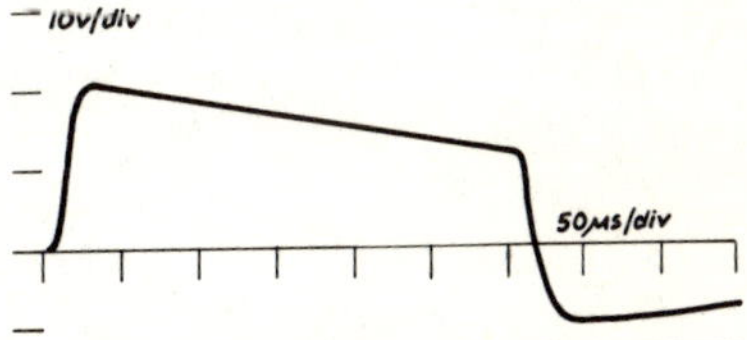

0.3ms	110Hz	22(44)into 1K 33 into 2K 38 into 3K 60(105) into 10K

Pos. 3 (treatment socket)

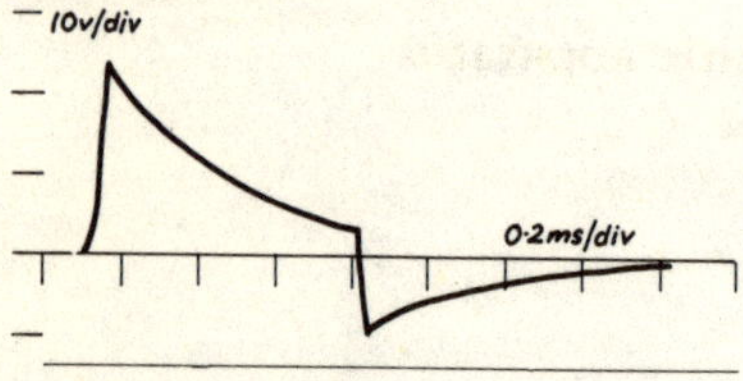

0.6ms	adjustable 0.8–90Hz	23(45) into 1K 34 into 2K 40 into 3K

Note. Figures above were taken with battery near to 1 volts/cell; the figures in brackets (where given) indicate output with a new battery at 1.5 volts/cell.

Pos. 3. (detection socket)
exploring point is always negative.

Skin resistance Kohms	*d.c. current mA*	*Audible frequency KHz*
0.2	1.35	3.8
1.0	1.3	4.2
2	1.2	4.5
5	1.0	5
10	0.7	6.3
20	0.4	8.7
Ultrasonic above this resistance value		
50	0.2	25

'frequency regulator' knob at max.

With knob set at 50 per cent some frequency stability sets in above 5 Kohms—squegging giving a lower frequency—not very reproducable.

Polarity

The Pink lead, positive on leading edge of all pulses, goes to the Auxiliary Point; while the negative goes to the Principal Point (manual).

Output Controls

Individual 4.7 Kohms potentiometers across each separate output transformer (primaries are driven in parallel).

Max. output resistance is about 1.3 Kohm at ½ max. output.

'Linearity' on 1 Kohm load

Dial	*Output Volts*
10	=48
8	=13
6	= 5
4	= 4
2	= 2
0	= 0

Control 'rough' between 9 and 10 (Patients usually treated between 4 and 8 on dial.)

Appendix II
Opium and heroin addiction: material and result

No.	*Age (yrs.)*	*Sex*	*Type of drug*	*Amount of drug (HK$/day)*	*Years of addic-tion*	*Diagnosis on admission*	*Response to treatment*	*Remarks*
1	50	M	Opium	$10	5	Concussion	Good	
2	72	M	Opium	$10	25	Chronic leg ulcer	Good	
3	62	M	Opium	$10	20	Fractured femur	Good	
4	64	M	Opium	$2	44	Pulmonary T.B. Chronic bronchitis	Good	
5	61	M	Opium	$10.20	40	Pulmonary emphysema	Good	Diarrhoea
6	65	M	Opium	$24	40	Rheumatism	Good	
7	69	M	Opium	$25	50	Low back pain	Good	
8	53	M	Opium	$6	3	Pulmonary T.B.	Good	
9	44	M	Opium	$8	29	Ashtma, Bronchitis	Good	
10	68	M	Opium	$10	51	Cor pulmonale	Good	
11	65	M	Opium	$30	42	Came for RX	Good	
12	51	M	Opium	$8	23	Concussion	Good	Urine test—doubtful
13	63	M	Opium	$10	33	Chronic bronchitis	Good	Low back pain
14	63	M	Opium	$5	32	Chronic bronchitis	Good	
15	55	M	Opium	$10	30	Skull fracture	Good	
16	69	M	Opium	$5	8	Chronic bronchitis	Good	Diarrhoea
17	66	M	Opium	$5	48	Atheroscerotic heart disease	Good	
18	60	M	Opium	$16	31	Cor pulmonale	Good	
19	50	M	Opium	$15	30	Chronic bronchitis	Good	
20	64	M	Opium	$5	46	Chronic bronchitis	Good	
21	56	M	Opium	$5	2	Cor pulmonale	Good	
22	60	M	Opium	$3	2	Chronic bronchitis	Good	
23	79	M	Opium	$30	58	Chronic bronchitis	Good	
24	60	M	Opium	$12	40	Tumour of bladder	—*	Urine test (+)
25	68	M	Opium	$10	46	Asthma, Bronchitis	Good	
26	56	M	Opium	$5	5	Asthma, Bronchitis	Good	
27	74	M	Opium	$3	20	Asthma, Bronchitis	Good	
28	60	M	Opium	$10	20	Pulmonary emphysema	Good	
29	65	M	Opium	$20	42	Pulmonary T.B.	Good	
30	57	M	Opium	$3	10	Pulmonary emphysema	Good	
31	60	M	Heroin	$30	35	Chronic bronchitis	Good	
32	54	M	Heroin	$30	27	Asthma, Bronchitis	Good	Frozen shoulder—right
33	43	M	Heroin	$15	15	Came for RX	Good	
34	58	M	Heroin	$25	15	Chronic bronchitis	Good	
35	44	M	Heroin	$20	15	Ankylosing spondylitis	Good	
36	17	F	Heroin	$20	2	Came for RX	Good	
37	22	M	Heroin	$40	2	Came for RX	Good	
38	29	M	Heroin	$30	3	Came for RX	Good	
39	43	M	Heroin	$10	12	Chronic bronchitis	Good	
40	38	M	Heroin	$5	12	Chronic bronchitis	Good	

* *Transferred to another hospital.*

Appendix III

Table 1. Clinical information on patients participating in study.

Case No.	*Age (Yrs.)*	*Sex*	*Duration of asthma (yrs.)*	*Admission in preceding 12 months (No.)*	*Previous short-term steroid therapy*	*Associated emphysema*	*Wdrst season*
1	65	M	3	8	?	*	Winter
2	49	M	6	8	Yes	*	,,
3	56	M	6	7	?	**	,,
4	14	F	9	5	Yes	*	,,
5	16	F	13	7	Yes	—	,,
6	15	F	9	4	Yes	—	,,

* *Mild to moderate emphysema*
** *Severe emphysema*

Table 2. Changes in pulmonary function values before and at ½ hour after acupuncture and electro-stimulation therapy for mild to moderate asthmatic attacks.

Case No.:		1	2	3	4	5	6
Associated Emphysema:		*	*	**	*	—	—
FEV1 (L)	Before	1.15	1.82	0.37	1.27	0.87	1.10
	After	1.65	2.30	0.47	1.90	1.72	1.50
FVC1 (L)	Before	2.10	3.95	1.12	2.25	1.92	1.63
	After	2.60	4.25	1.20	2.60	2.10	1.83
FEV1/FVC (%)	Before	54.8	46.1	33.0	56.4	45.3	67.5
	After	63.5	54.1	39.2	73.1	81.9	82.0
PEFR (L/Min)	Before	200	280	60	120	134	135
	After	304	372	92	226	212	185

* *Mild to moderate emphysema*
** *Severe emphysema*

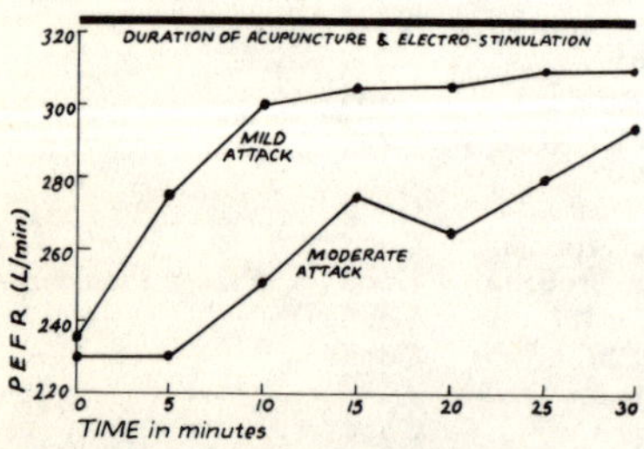

Fig. 1. The change in PEFR in one patient during acupuncture and electro-stimulation therapy for two separate asthmatic attacks. Note difference in time of onset of response.

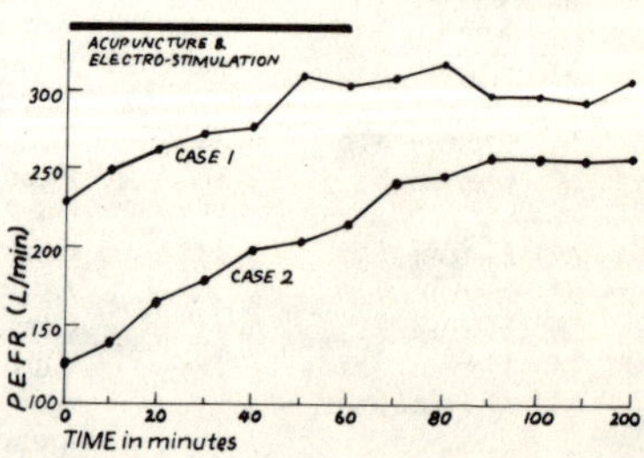

Fig. 2. The change in PEFR in two patients during acupuncture and electro-stimulation therapy for moderately severe asthmatic attacks. Note PEFR continues to rise after cessation of therapy

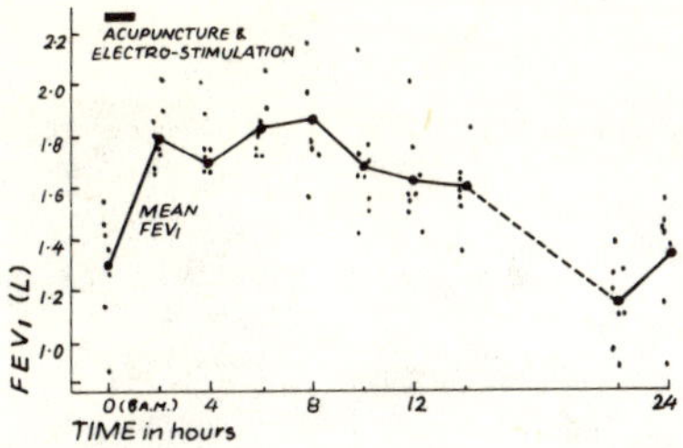

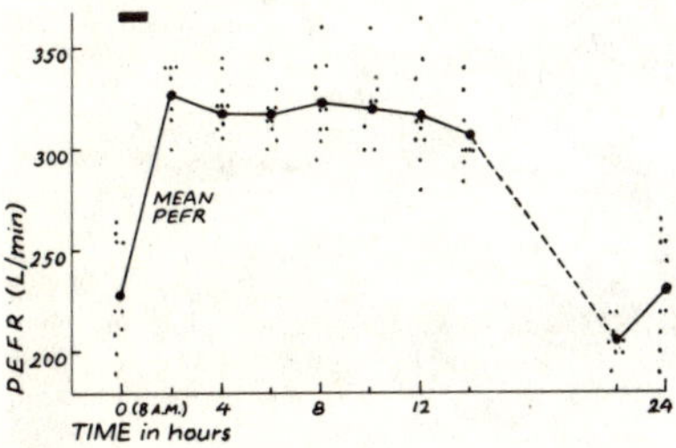

Fig. 3a and Fig. 3b. The change in serial measurements of FEV1 and PEFR respectively in a patient with severe bronchial asthma (case 1) over a 10-day period during which the bronchial asthma was treated solely by acupuncture and electro-stimulation therapy. (One session of acupuncture and electro-stimulation from 45 min. to one hour was given at 8 a.m. every morning (0 hour). Significant improvement of mean FEV1 and PEFR was recorded after therapy and was maintained relatively well throughout the day. No recording was made during sleep. Symptomatically, the patient had good clinical response and was symptom-free most of the time. He commented that he was subjectively better during this period than when he was on conventional therapy. By the conclusion of the present report, he was maintained successfully on this regimen for four weeks.)

Table 3. Clinical response to acupuncture and electro-stimulation therapy during asthmatic attacks.

Severity of asthmatic attack	*Time of onset of effect*	*Time of relief of distress*	*Duration of relief*
Mild	3-5 min.	5-15 min.	10-24 hrs.
Moderate to severe	10-15 min.	30-60 min.	4-12 hrs.
Very severe	½-2 hrs.	1-4 hrs.	1-6 hrs.

Table 4. Reduction of daily oral bronchodilator dosage in patients on follow-up treatment with acupuncture and electro-stimulation.

Case No.		2	4	5	6
Doses of oral bronchodilator daily	Previous	3	4	4	3
	After acupuncture and electro-stimulation therapy	0-2	2-3	1	1

Appendix IV

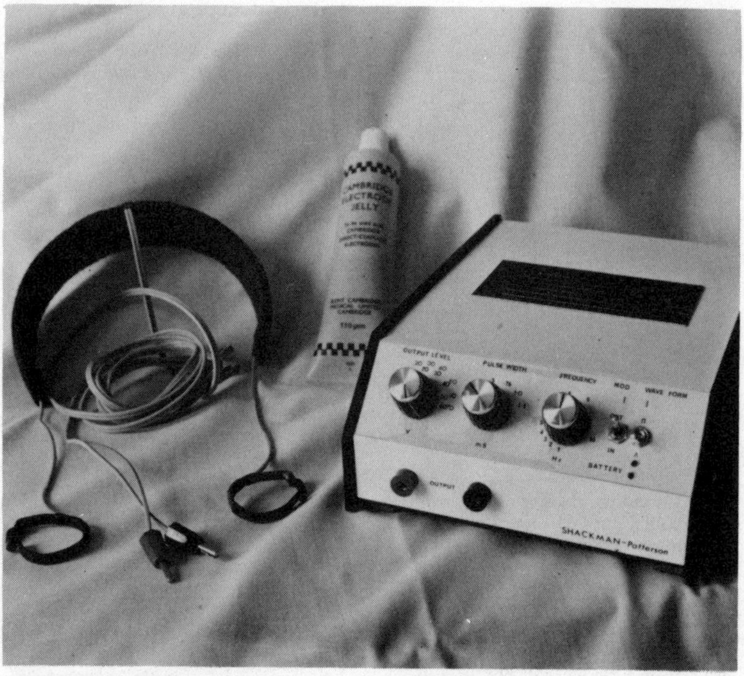

Shackman-Patterson electrical stimulator

Actual size: $8\frac{1}{2}$ x $5\frac{5}{8}$ x 3 in., and wt. (including batteries) $3\frac{1}{2}$ lbs. (1.59 kilo). Produces a rectangular or peaked wave-form, with or without modulation of 50KHz. Variable frequency of 5-2000Hz (cps). Variable pulse width of 0.1-1.5 msecs (the chart which is permanently attached to the upper surface of the machine shows the precise frequency relative to various pulse-widths). There is no distortion of the wave-form on changing frequency. The voltage is completely independent and has an output of 0/60 volts peak to peak into a 1K ohm load. Batteries: 2 x PP1 (or equivalent). Can also be supplied with 4 outputs for simultaneous use, and/or with a built-in timer. The headband may be worn on the head, or sit at the back of the neck, whichever the patient finds most comfortable. Can be used with blunt ear electrodes (incorporated in a head-set) for addictions to drugs, alcohol and nicotine and related conditions. Electrode jelly should be applied to electrodes. Can also be used with distal electrodes for pain but generalized pain can sometimes be helped by using ear electrodes.

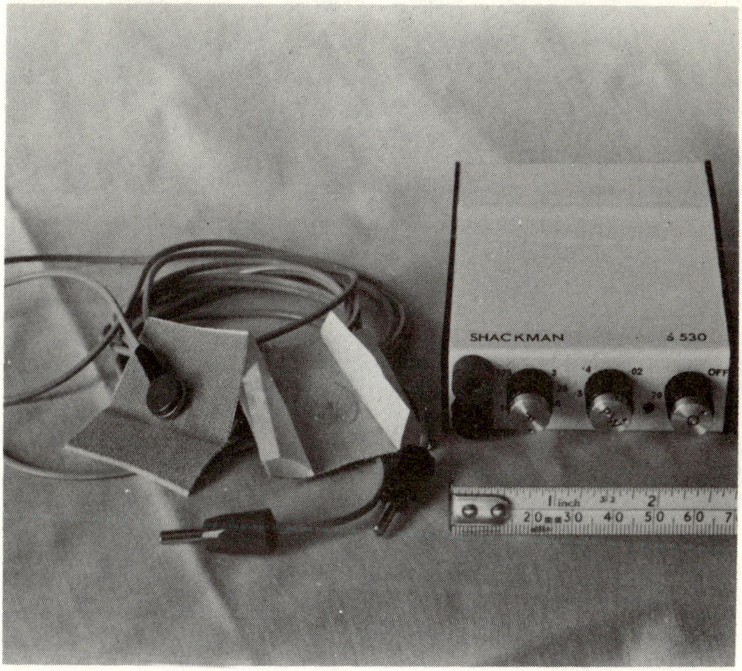

Pocket-size stimulator S530

Portable model for use mainly in pain. Actual size 4 x 3 x $1\frac{3}{8}$ in. and wt. $9\frac{1}{2}$ oz. (0.28 kilo). Rectangular wave-form only: variable frequency 3-125Hz (cps) and pulse width 0.04 to 0.4 msecs. Variable output 0-70 volts into a 1K ohm load. Batteries 4 x HP7 (or equivalent). Can be supplied with rechargeable batteries and battery charger. Press-stud electrodes for connection to any standard electrodes (adhesive plaster ellectrodes in illustration); crocodile clip connecting leads also available. (Machines designed by Shackman Instruments Ltd., Chesham, England.)

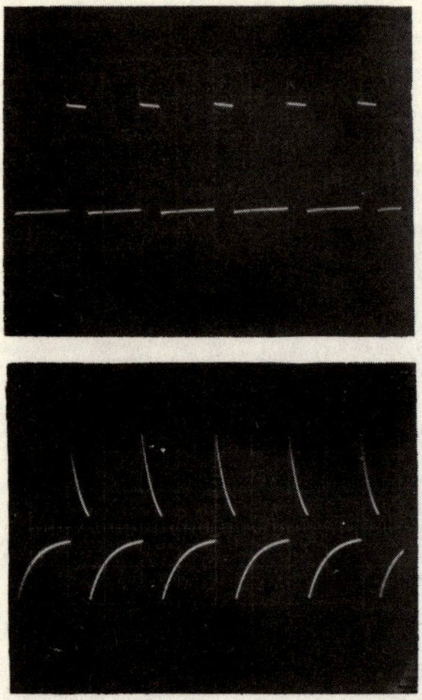

Top, square and *above*, spiked wave forms.

Frequency: 1KHz, 0.25 msec pulse width. Time base: 0.5 msec/cm (horizontal), and Y amplitude: 20v pp/cm (vertical).

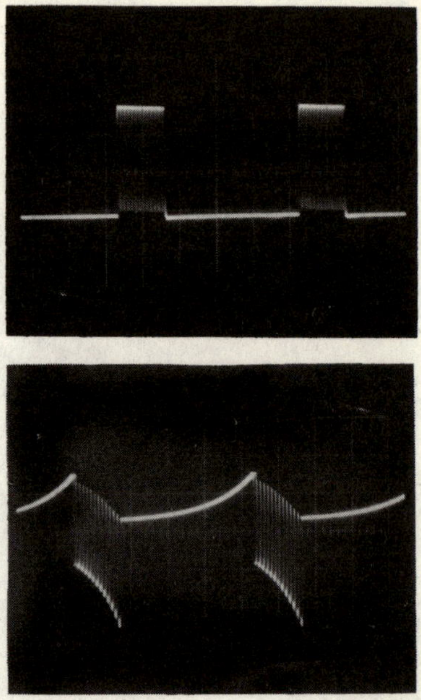

Top, square and *above*, spiked modulated wave forms.

Frequency: 1KHz, 0.25 msec pulse width. Time base: 0.2 msec/cm (horizontal) and Y amplitude: 20v pp/cm (vertical).

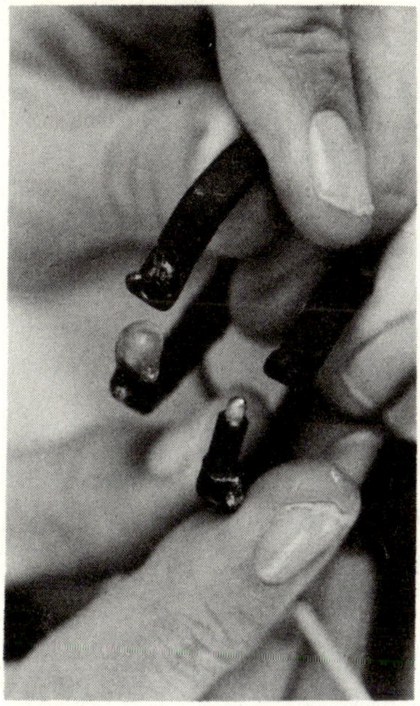

Close-up of ear-electrodes. They are entirely insulated except for the metal tip, and can be bent to exert the correct amount of pressure. A blob of electrode jelly is placed on the metal tip, to give a smooth conduction of the current.

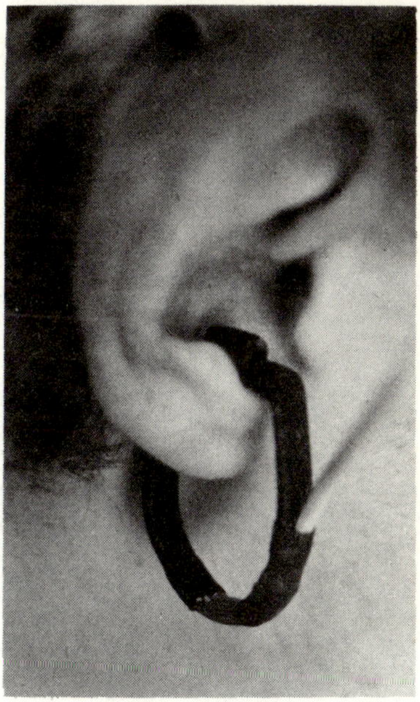

Close-up of electrode in position on the ear. The metal tip is placed in the concha.